I0478391

RCE GROUP USA
3:03
Mother
Father
1:34
4:39
2:19
ncellab
1:13
1:12
SEMDCSA
SOUTH EAST SEMDCSA, LLC
www.SEMDCSA.com
2:34
PharmRCC
4:14
3:36
3:22

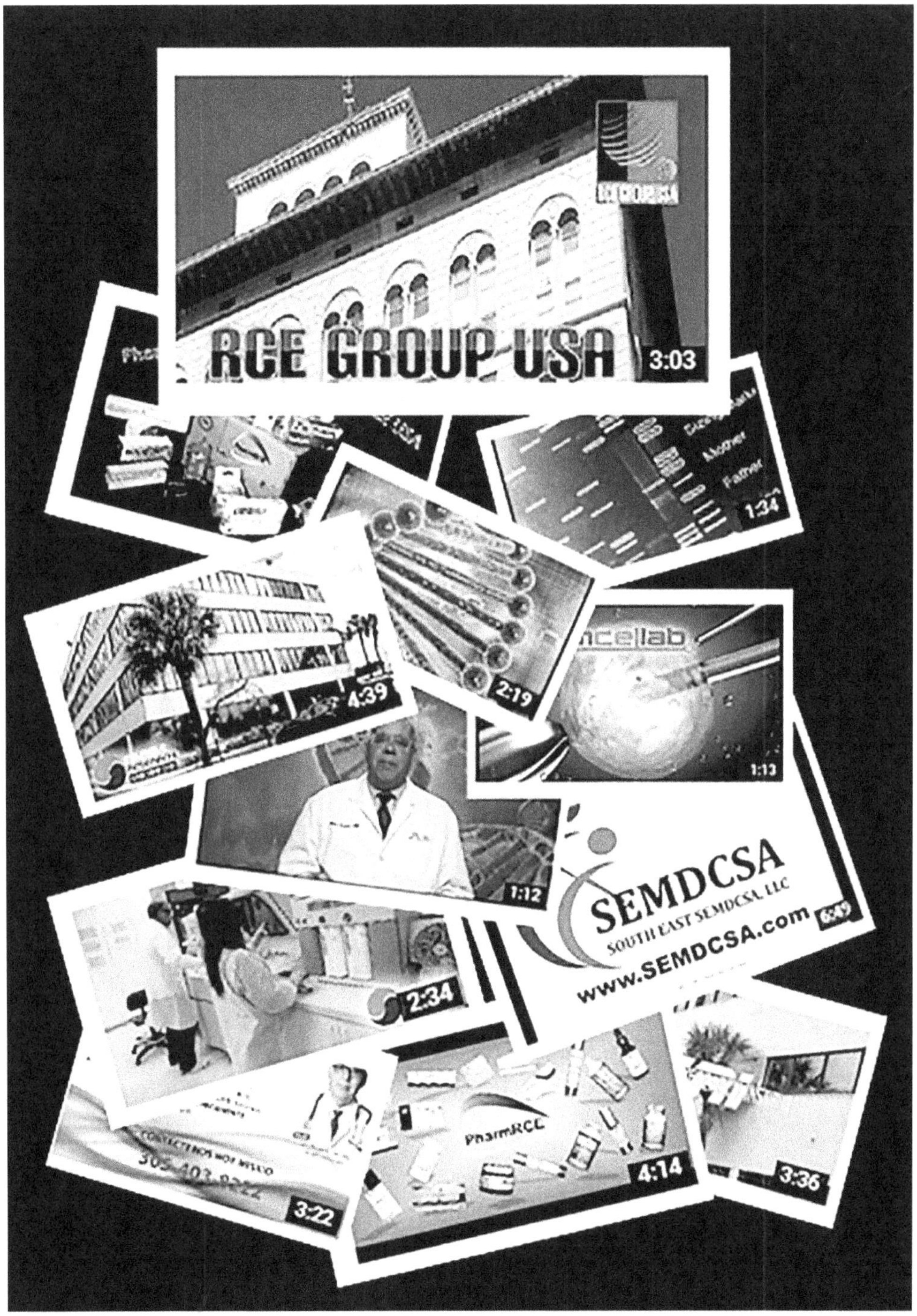

INDICE

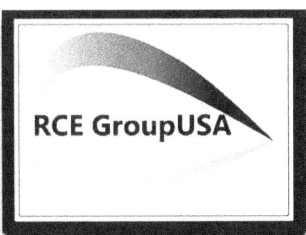
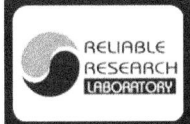
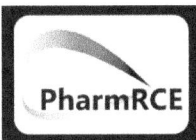
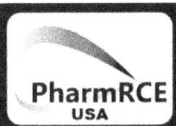
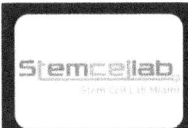
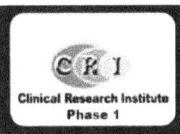
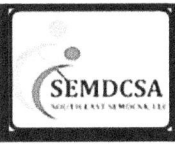

INTRODUCCION

RCE Group USA, es un conglomerado de empresas y/o entidades que ha servido en el Campo de la Salud por más de 25 años. Está conformado un grupo polivalente que abarca diferentes campos de la medicina y la farmacología, tales como los aspectos Clínicos, Educación para posgraduados de carreras médicas, Investigaciones farmacéuticas, Aspectos de la cosmetología y cuidado de la piel, Temas relacionados con el uso de las Células madres, entre otras cosas.

RCE Group USA bajo la dirección general del Dr. Hugo Romeu. M.D. y tiene la ventaja que acopia bajo la misma sombrilla, las diversas aristas necesarias para viabilizar cualquier proyecto relacionado con el campo de la salud. La experiencia del Dr. Romeu en el campo integral de la medicina, es uno de los aspectos más relevantes y valioso de nuestro grupo, más de 30 años trabajando día a día de manera prolija como especialista patólogo y liderando más de 700 estudios de investigación farmacéutica, aspectos como estos hacen del Dr. Romeu una pieza clave, debido a su dedicación, experiencia y reconocimientos múltiples en diversos países, dentro esta especialidad.

RCE Group USA, ha trabajado conjuntamente con científicos diseñadores de múltiples países, con vistas a la obtención de dichas acreditaciones, motivo por el cual goza de un prestigio mundial en esta gestión. Adicionalmente a las corporaciones que forman la estructura de nuestro equipo de trabajo, nuestro grupo está asociado a diversas empresas a manera de Empresas conjuntas, Joint Ventures, logrando de este modo, adicionar fluidez y profesionalismo al desarrollo de cualquier proyecto sin importar la envergadura del mismo.

Le invitamos a que conozca nuestro grupo y nuestra disposición de serle útil de inmediato en cualquier proyecto relacionado con el abanico de proyecciones que dominan nuestros expertos.

Dr. Hugo Romeu M.D.

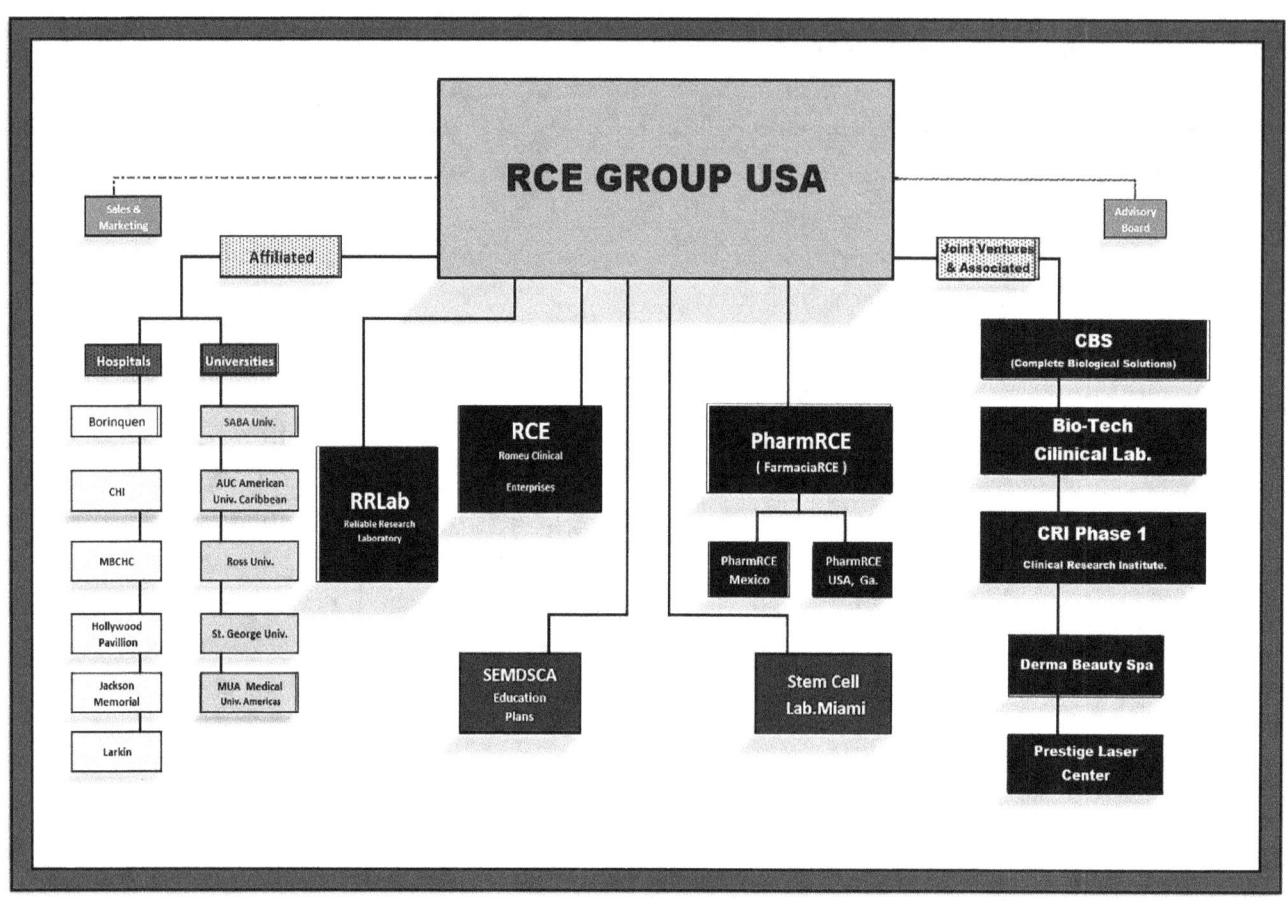

ORGANIGRAMA RCE GROUP USA

RCE Group USA
Dr. Hugo Romeu M.D.

RCE GROUP USA

dr.hugoromeu@yahoo.com

RCE Group USA

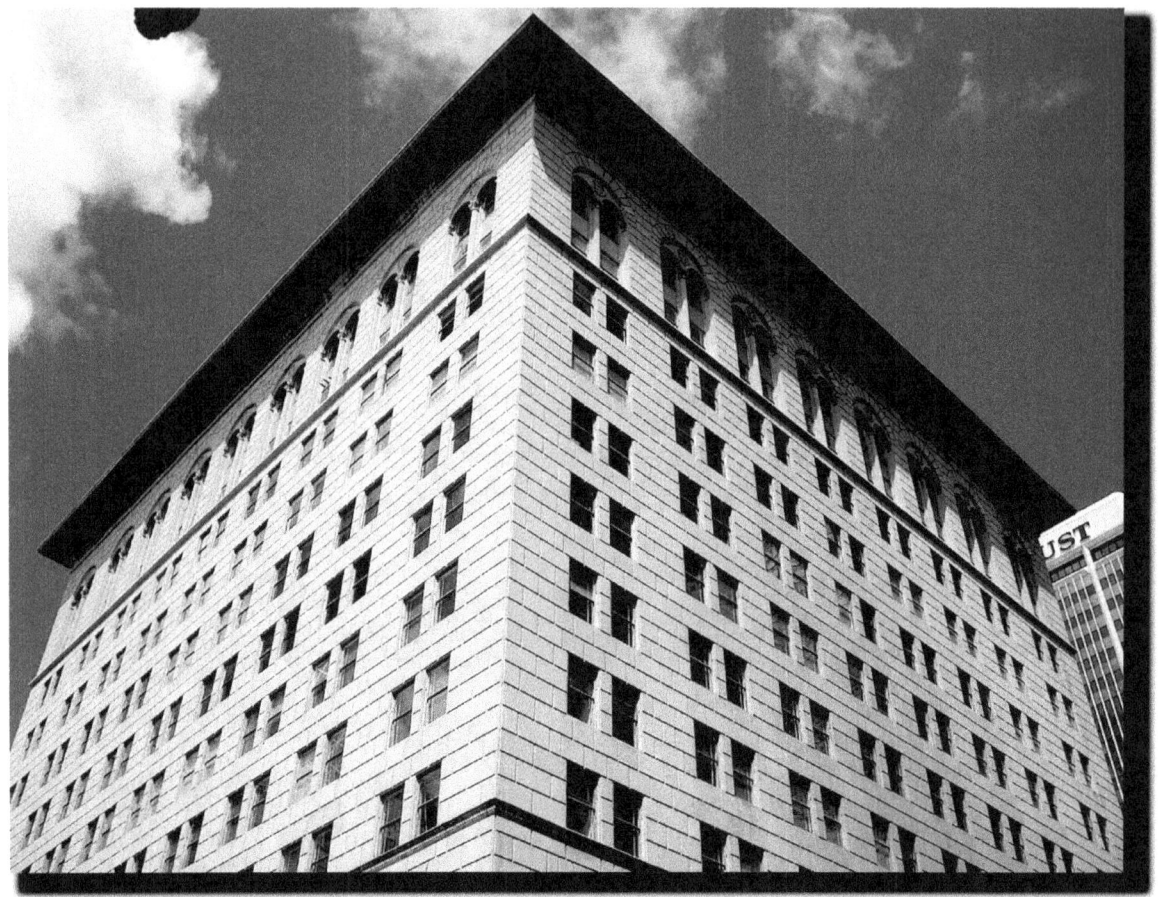

Ingraham Building
25 Southeast Second Avenue, Suite 818. Miami, Fl, 33131
Phone: (305) 642 7011 Fax: (305) 642 0772
www.RCEGroupUSA.com

RCE Group USA, es un conglomerado de empresas y/o entidades que ha servido en el Campo de la Salud por más de 25 años.

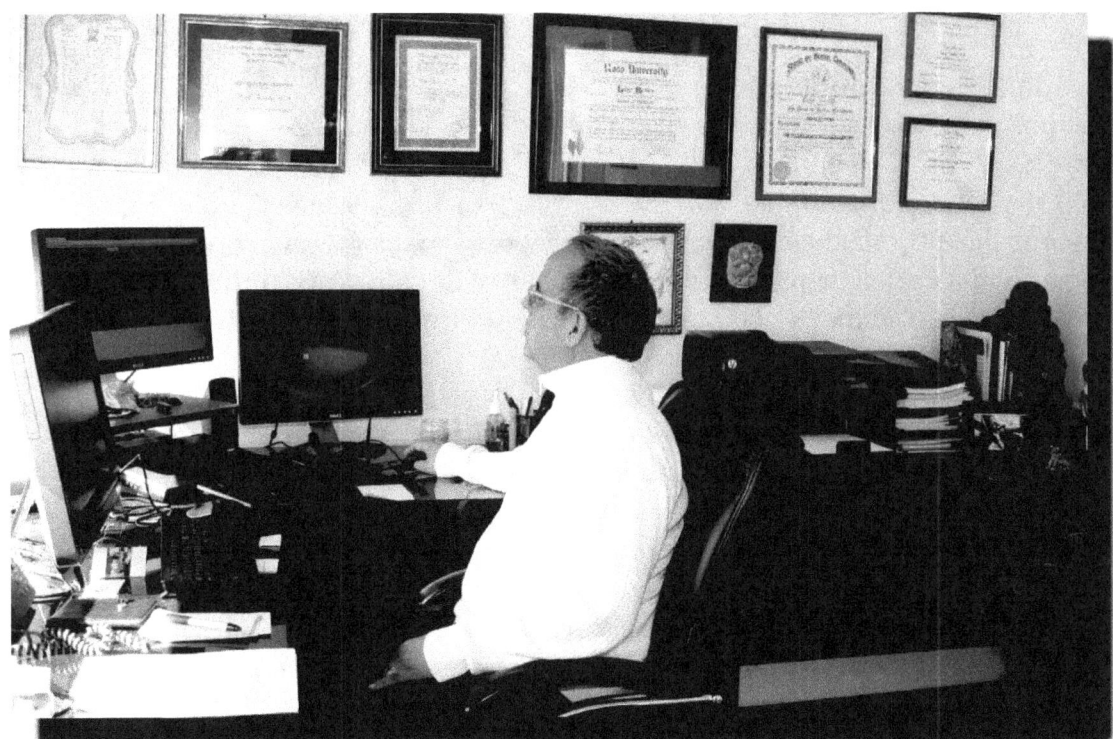

Dr. Hugo Romeu. M.D.

RCE Group USA, es un grupo polivalente que abarca diferentes campos de la medicina, tales como los aspectos Clínicos, Educación para posgraduados decarreras médicas , Investigaciones farmacéuticas, Aspectos de la cosmetología y cuidado de la piel, Temas relacionados con el uso de las Células madres y todo lo relacionado con el campo de la farmacología.

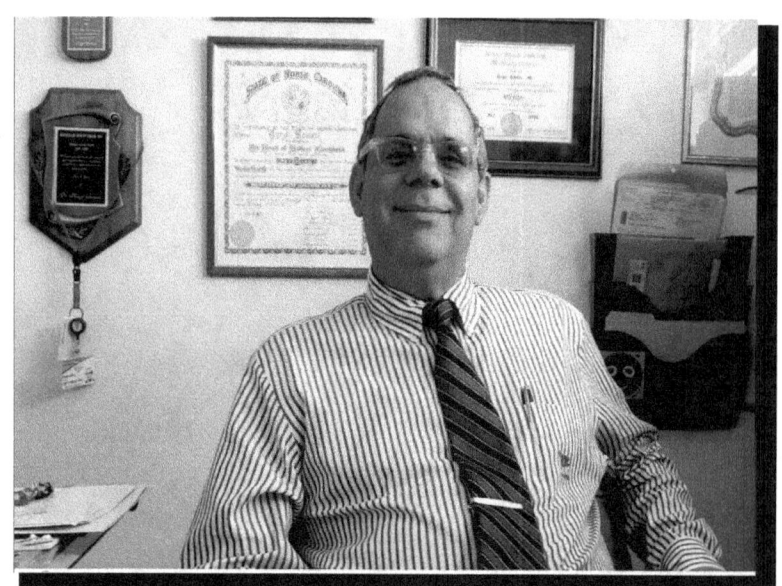

RCE Group USA bajo la dirección general del *Dr. Hugo Romeu. M.D.* tiene la ventaja que acopia bajo la misma sombrilla, las diversas aristas necesarias para viabilizar cualquier proyecto relacionado con el campo de la salud.

La experiencia del *Dr. Romeu* en el campo integral de la medicina, es uno de los aspectos más relevantes y valioso de nuestro grupo, más de 30 años trabajando día a día de manera prolija como especialista patólogo y liderando más de 700 estudios de investigación farmacéutica, aspectos como estos hacen del *Dr. Romeu* una pieza clave, debido a su dedicación, experiencia y reconocimientos múltiples en diversos países dentro

esta especialidad.

El supremo mandato de la *FDA* es regular la multitud de productos medicinales de tal manera que proteja la seguridad de los consumidores estadounidenses y la efectividad de los medicamentos comercializados. El presupuesto de la *FDA* para aprobar, etiquetar y controlar medicamentos es de unos 290 millones de dólares al año. Los *"Equipos de Revisión"* emplean alrededor de 1,900 empleados que evalúan los nuevos medicamentos. El *"Equipo de Seguridad"* cuenta con 72 empleados para determinar si un nuevo medicamento es inseguro o presenta riesgos no declarados en la ficha técnica del producto.

El Equipo de Seguridad controla los efectos de más de 3000 medicamentos de venta con receta sobre una población de 200 millones de personas con un presupuesto de $15 millones de dólares. La *FDA* requiere que cada nuevo medicamento sea evaluado a través de una serie sucesiva de 4 fases de ensayos clínicos, siendo la fase 3 la más extensa, y en la que se realizan pruebas en 1,000 a 3,000 pacientes.

Un medicamento que después de haber sido probado y haber mostrado sus cualidades, que además esta bien diseñado y elaborado, puede ser que obtenga ciertos

logros de distribución y venta en ciertos escenarios, pero cuando ese producto ha sido certificado y acreditado por la *FDA*, para su distribución y venta
en los *Estados Unidos*, sin duda tiene el éxito garantizado.

RCE Group USA, está en la capacidad de dirigir y elaborar los protocolos necesarios, con vistas a obtener los permisos y las pautas, que den inicio a una
investigación farmacéutica con el rigor y las exigencias de los organismos gubernamentales de los Estados Unidos.

Estos pasos son necesarios para lograr eventualmente la aprobación y/o acreditación de la *FDA (Food and Drugs Administration)*, para cada medicamento en específico, esa calificación es absolutamente necesaria para la
comercialización de dicho medicamento en los Estados Unidos.

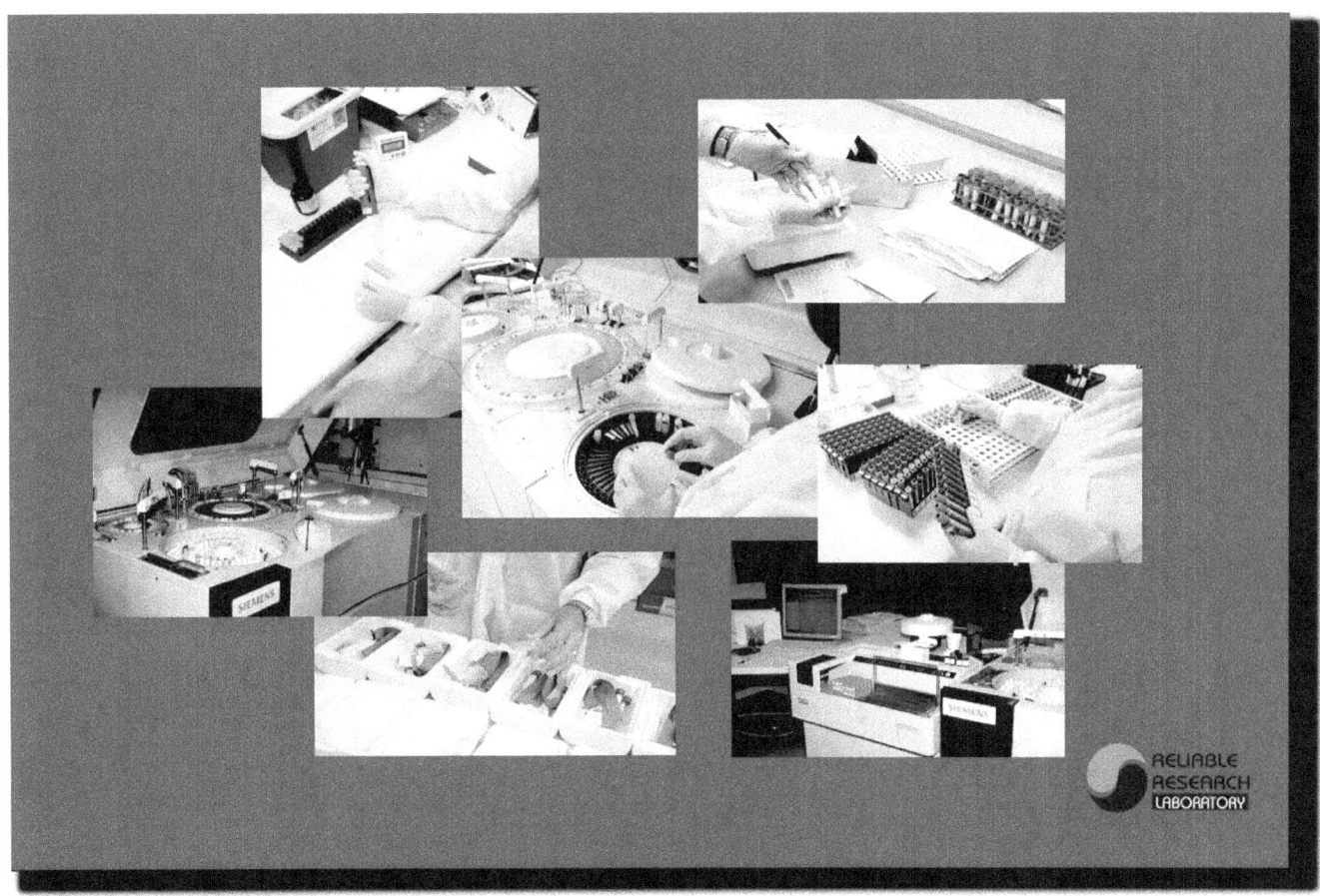

RCE Group USA, ha trabajado conjuntamente con los científicos diseñadores de múltiples países, con vistas a la obtención de dichas acreditaciones, motivo por el cual goza de un prestigio mundial en esta gestión.

Adicionalmente a las corporaciones que forman la estructura de nuestro equipo de trabajo, nuestro grupo está asociado a diversas empresas a manera *de Joint Ventures*, logrando de este modo, adicionar fluidez y profesionalismo al desarrollo de cualquier proyecto, ya que la dependencia de agentes exteriores, en la mayoría de los casos se hace innecesaria.

RCE Group USA, cuenta con un Laboratorio especializado en investigaciones *Reliable Research laboratory,* con un equipamiento de la más alta tecnología, con profesionales y técnicos altamente calificados, que sumados sobrepasan más de cien años de experiencia. Este laboratorio con más de 20 años de trabajo, abarca todas las fases de la industria farmacéutica.

También contamos con un centro de investigaciones, *CRI (Clinical research Institute),* que ha llevado a cabo múltiples estudios en diversas capacidades, ya sea en las fases iniciales, *Phase 1,* u otras etapas de la investigación como las *Phase 2, 3 y 4.* Este Instituto cuenta con especialistas de la más alta calificación.

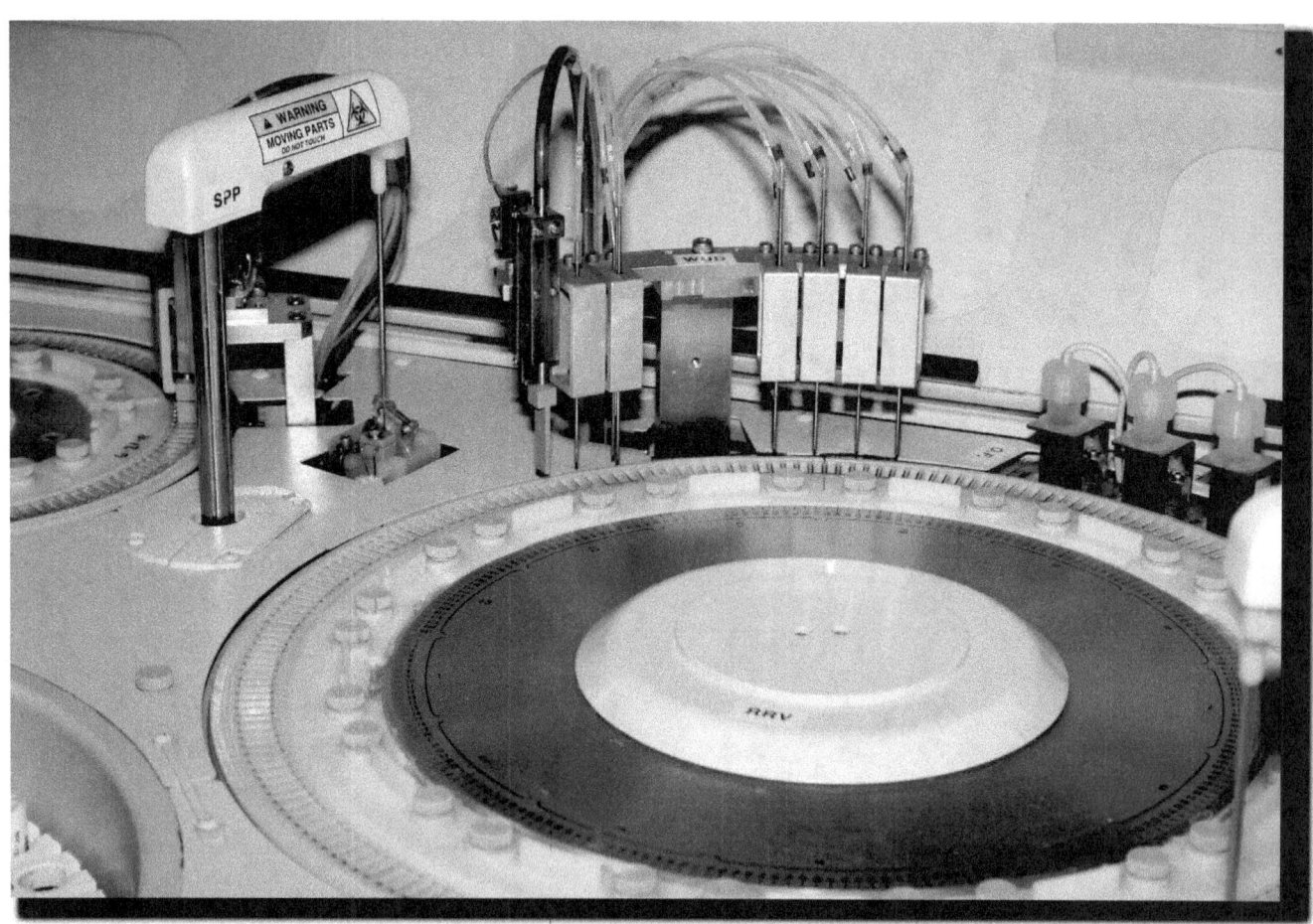

RCE Group USA, tiene una dependencia dedicada por entero al campo de la farmacia, esta empresa *PharmRCE* atiende todo lo relacionado con la distribución de medicamentos y equipos médicos. Estamos en la capacidad de enviar a cualquier sitio, un pedido personal de veinte dólares o un pedido comercial de un millón de dólares, la única limitación será la capacidad de los fabricantes de honrarnos nuestros pedidos.

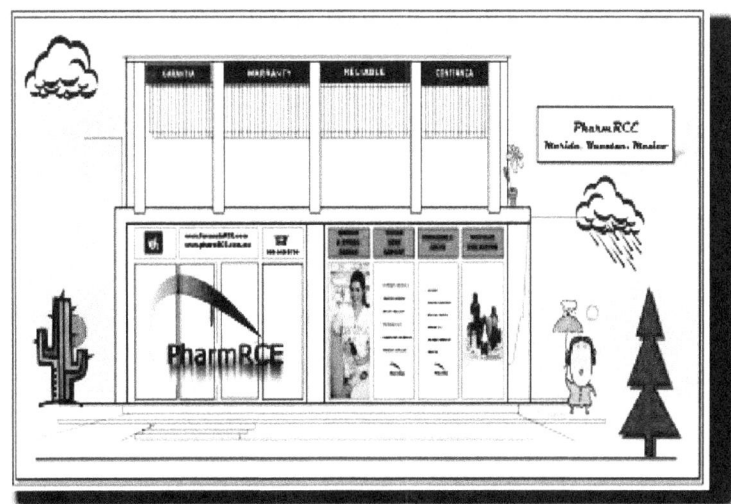

Nuestra empresa, con base en Mérida, Yucatán. México, posee la infraestructura necesaria, para Exportar, Importar o distribuir medicamentos a diferentes destinos.

Estamos capacitados para proceder al envió inmediato de medicamentos a familiares donde quiera que estos se encuentren, con pedidos que se pueden ordenar desde cualquier parte del mundo, incluyendo los Estados Unidos.

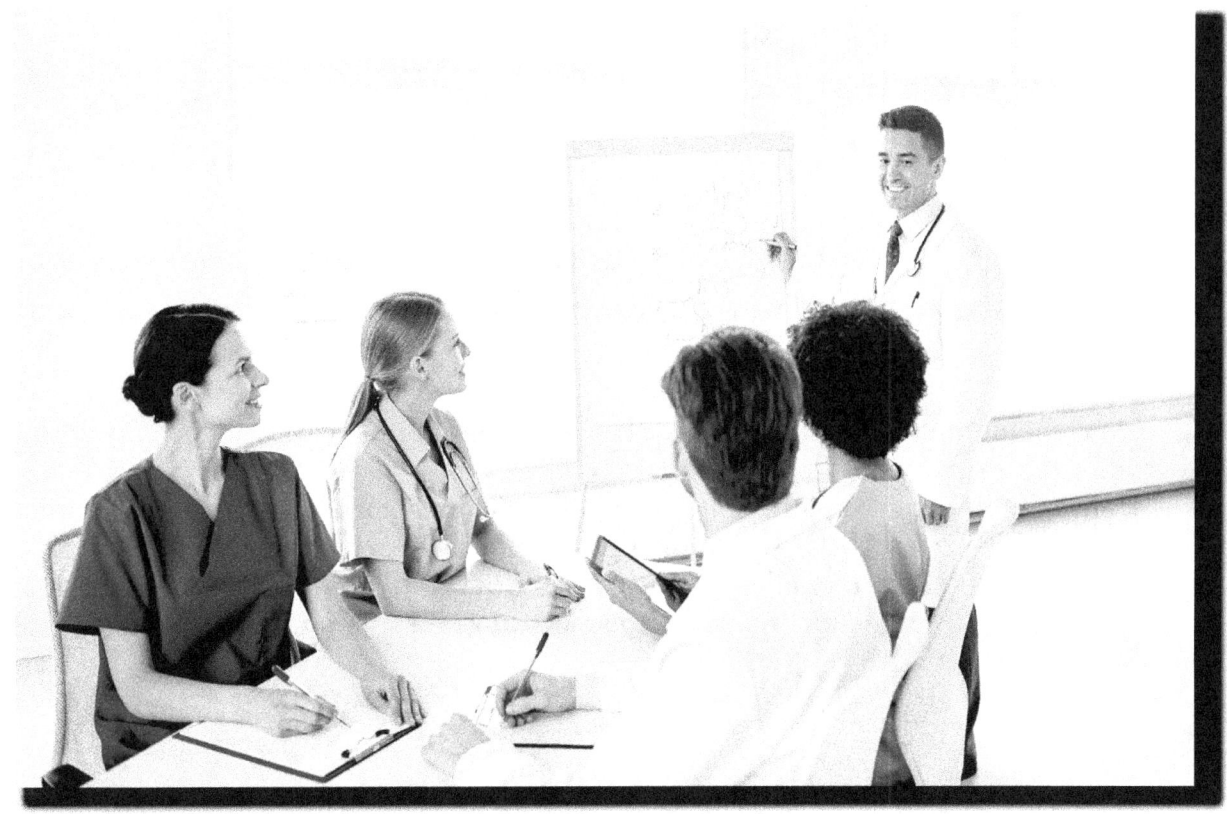

Romeu Clinical Enterprises, está envuelto en la formación profesional de estudiantes y graduados de las diferentes escuelas de medicinas tanto en el país como fuera de este.

Nuestro propósito es facilitar las diferentes rotaciones necesarias para la obtención de las más altas acreditaciones como la ACGME.

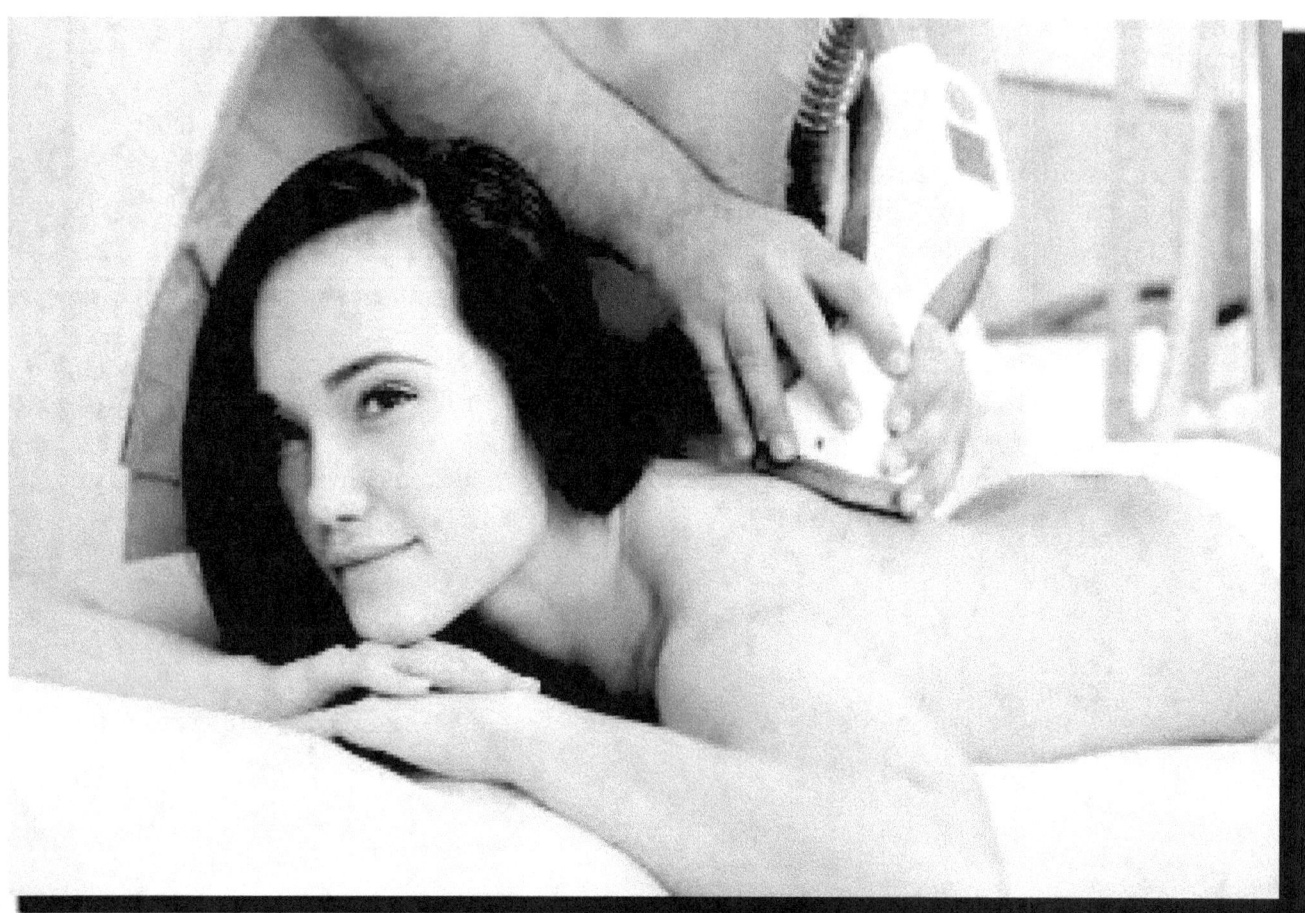

Hasta el momento han pasado por nuestros entrenamientos y rotaciones más de 1,200 estudiantes y graduados de medicina.

Hemos incursionado en el diseño en la elaboración de fórmulas relativas al cuidado de la piel. *Derma Beauty Spa*, es un centro de embellecimiento y tratado de la piel que contempla los principales servicios en esa área y aplica la extraordinaria experiencia del *Dr. Romeu* en ese campo, como lo muestra su libro *"Beauty & Skin. Reflexion in health care"*.

Por otro lado **Prestige Laser Center**, es un centro con una
muy elevada tecnología relativa al uso del láser en la eliminación o reducción de
aspectos indeseados que
facilitan el alcance de la belleza, con la más alta tecnología y con un personal
altamente calificado.

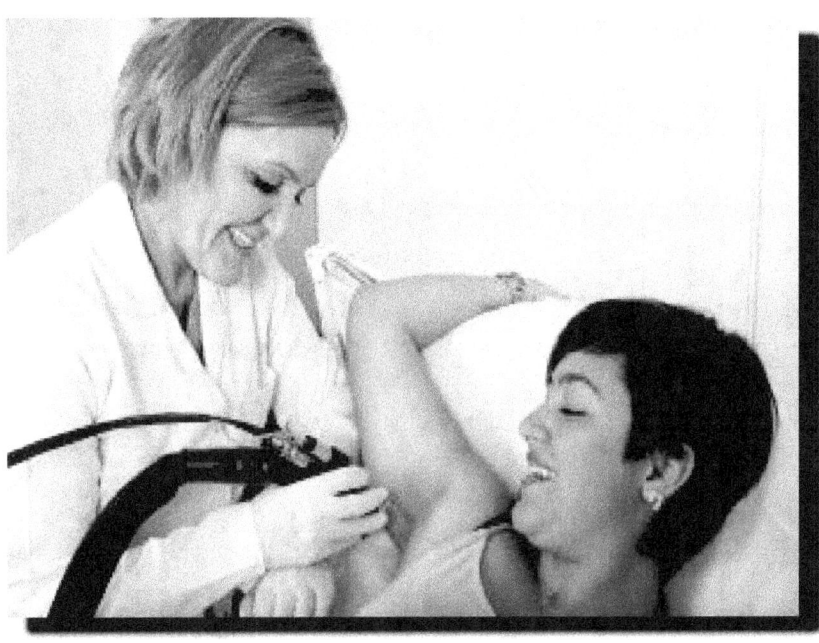

RCE Group USA, ha incursionado en el campo del uso de las Células Madres. **STEAM CELL LAB** es un laboratorio de células madres privado que trabaja en
equipo con una clínica de investigación fiable.

Nuestro equipo de científicos ha estado trabajando por más de 25 años al servicio de establecimientos de salud, sitios de atención primaria y clínicas de todos los diferentes
tamaños, además de los hospitales y de la industria farmacéutica.
Hemos completado más de 700 investigaciones que atienden a las peticiones de casi
cada empresa farmacéutica.

Muchos son los planes de ampliación de la capacidad de nuestro grupo, siempre dirigidas a hacer más universal y eficiente nuestra gestión.

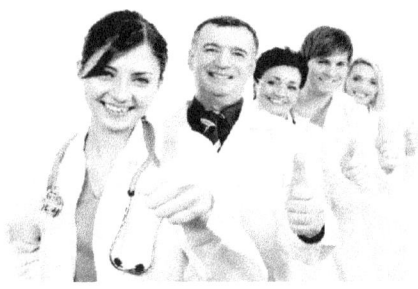

RCE Group USA les invita a visitar sus instalaciones e intercambiar con su personal, con vistas a usar nuestros servicios para llevar a cabo sus proyectos.

Juntos haremos la diferencia.

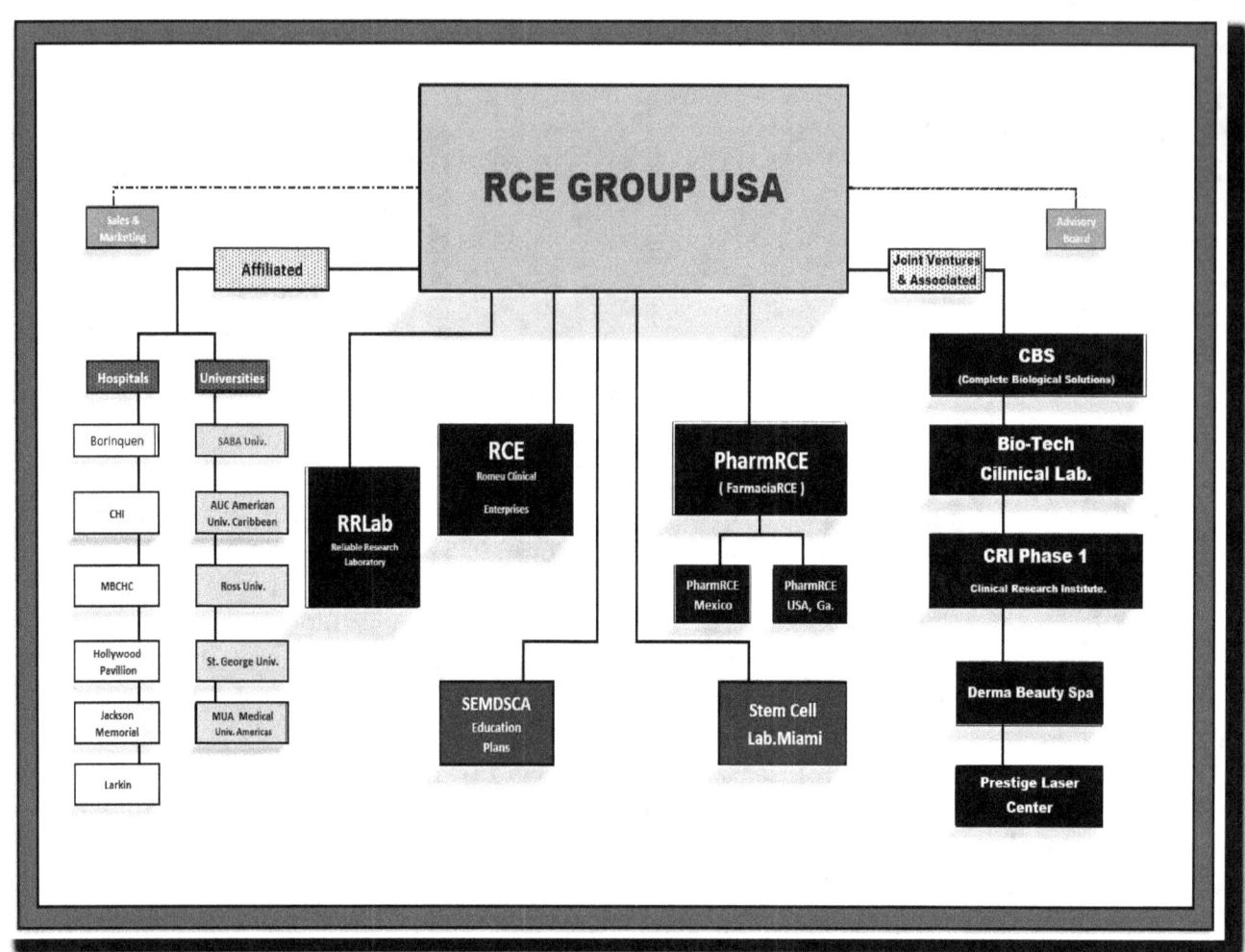

ORGANIGRAMA RCE GROUP USA

HUGO ROMEU, MD

Médico General – Médico Cirujano – Médico Patólogo

Licenciado en el Estado de la Florida: ME64804

(305)281 36 33 – (305)642 70 11

dr.hugoromeu@yahoo.com

Breve reseña de la experiencia en el campo de la medicina del Doctor Hugo Romeu.

EXPERIENCIA

Reliable Research Laboratory (Miami, FL), 2013 – Present
Director Médico – Patólogo – Responsable de Operaciones del Laboratorio Clínico – Revisión de Procedimientos de Laboratorio – Oficiar Reuniones de Control de Calidad – Pruebas de Aptitud – Cumplir con los Deberes establecidos por CLIA, Cola y CAP.

Romeu Clinical Enterprises (Miami, FL), 1995 – Presente
Director Ejecutivo de Operaciones – Director Médico.

Phase One Solution (Miami, FL), 2012 – 2013
Socio Administrativo, Director Ejecutivo de Operaciones, Director Médico.

PRACS Institute (Miami, FL), 2012 – 2013
Director Médico – Patólogo – Responsable de Operaciones del Laboratorio Clínico – Revisión de Procedimientos de Laboratorio – Oficiar Reuniones de Control de Calidad – Pruebas de Aptitud – Cumplir con los Deberes establecidos por CLIA, Cola y CAP.

Cetero Research (Miami, FL), 2009 – 2012
Director Médico – Patólogo – Responsable de Operaciones del Laboratorio Clínico – Revisión de Procedimientos de Laboratorio Anualmente – Oficiar Reuniones de Control de Calidad – Pruebas de Aptitud – Cumplir con los Deberes establecidos por CLIA, Cola y CAP.

Allied Research International (Miami, FL), 2006 – 2009
Director Médico – Patólogo – Responsable de Operaciones del Laboratorio Clínico – Revisión de Procedimientos de Laboratorio – Oficiar Reuniones de Control de Calidad – Pruebas de Aptitud – Cumplir con los Deberes establecidos por CLIA, Cola y CAP.

SFBCI (Miami, FL), 2001 – 2006
Director Médico – Patólogo – Responsable de Operaciones del Laboratorio Clínico – Revisión de Procedimientos de Laboratorio – Oficiar Reuniones de Control de Calidad – Pruebas de Aptitud – Equipo de Médicos Patólogos – Investigador - Cumplir con los Deberes establecidos por CLIA, Cola y CAP.

American Health Associates (Hialeah, FL), 2000 – 2005
Director de Laboratorio.

Gatewa y Laboratory (Pompano, FL), 1998 – 2001
Director Médico – Personal Médico de Patología.

Biotrace Laboratories (Miami, FL), 1996 – 1998
Director Médico - Personal Médico de Patología – Cirugía Patológica – Citología.

Center of Laboratory Medicine (Miami, FL), 1993 – 1996
Director Médico - Personal Médico de Patología – Cirugía Patológica – Citología

Florida Keys Pathology (Miami, FL), 1993 – 1994
Personal Médico de Patología – Cirugía Patológica – Citología
Ho l l y w o o d D i a g n os t i c C e nt e r (Hollywood, FL), 1990 – 1993. Director Médico - Personal Médico de Patología.

U.S 5 th General Hospital (Stuttgart, West Germany), 1986 – 1990. Personal Médico de Patología – Cirugía Patológica – Citología – Investigación.

Cook Count y Institute of Forensic Science (Chicago, IL),
1984– 86. Director Médico - Personal Médico de Patología

EDUCACION

HIGH SCHOOL DIPLOMA:
Loyola Academy (Wilmette, IL), 1969 – 1973

PRE -MEDICAL :
Loyola University (Chicago, IL – Rome Italy), 1973 – 1976

DOCTOR OF MEDICINE :
Ross University of NY (New York, NY), 1976 – 1980

PGY 1 & 2 ANATOMIA PATOLOGICA :
State University of NY (New York, NY), 1980 – 1982

PGY 3 ANATOMIA PATOLOGICA:
Saint Joseph's Hospital (Milwaukee, WI), 1982 – 1983

PGY 4 PATOLOGICA FORENSE:
Cook County Institute of Forensic Science (Chicago, IL), 1983 – 1984

PEDIATRIA PATOLOGICA:
Children's Memorial Hospital (Buffalo, NY), 1981 – 1982

PATOLOGIC A DE TUMOR :
Roswell Park Memorial Insitute (Buffalo, NY), 1981 – 1981

CITPATOLOGIA:
Saint Joseph's Hospital (Milwaukee, WI), 1983 – 1984

PATOLOGICA FORENSE:
Cook & Eric County Medical Examiner (Chicago, IL), 1983 – 1984

MICROSCOPIO ELECTRON:
Buffalo General Hospital (Buffalo, NY), 1980 – 1982

PROYECTOS ESPECIALE S

COLABORACION : Alemania 1 9 8 5
Con especialistas del instituto de endocrinología de La Habana en Alemania Occidental en la Investigación de Diabetes Tipo I y II

INVESTIGAC ION : La Habana, Cuba, 1985-86
En el Instituto de Endocrinología en la Habana, Sala Gordon, Hospital Calixto García.

COLABORACION : La Habana, Cuba, 1985-87
En el Instituto de Oncología en la Habana.

GALARDON : La Habana, Cuba, 1987
Mejor trabajo científico del año 1986 en estos proyectos.

MODERNIZACION : Checoslovaquia, 1980-90
De sistemas computarizados para laboratorios clínicos.

INSTALACION : Hungría, 1985-90 de sistemas de información para las computadoras de Laboratorios Clínicos.

INVESTIGACION : La Habana, Cuba, 1987

Microangiopatia Renal, Respuesta Auto-Inmune, Proyecto de Investigación en la Universidad de la Habana.

INVESTIGACION : La Habana, Cuba, 1987

Herpes Virus Encefalitis, La Ultra Estructura se Vuelve útil en el diagnóstico. Proyecto de Investigación en la Universidad de la Habana.

INVESTIGACION : Chicago,IL 1984-1987

Investigación y Estudio Forense de "Atípicas Heridas de Bala" en la Oficina del Medico Examinador de Cook County.

DISCURSOS Y PUBLICACIONES

INTRODUCCION: Saint Kittens (U.S Virgin Island) 2015

A la ceremonia de graduación de Médicos de la Universidad de Medicina y Ciencias de la Salud de Saint Kittens (U.M.H.S.)

DISCURSO: Harvard, 2015. De iniciación ante los estudiantes de Medicina HARVARD MEDICAL SCHOOL.

AUTOR: 2015 Libro "Skin Secrets, The practical approach to looks younger"   ("Secretos de la Piel, una aproximación practica a verse mas joven") y Libro "Skin Secrets, The practical approach to looks younger" 2015.

"Embolia de Gas Arterial Relacionado con Contaminación de Monóxido de Carbón" Presentado al Periódico de Ciencia Forense. 1994

"El Fenómeno Autoinmune en Conversión a la Diabetes Tipo II en
 la Variante Dependiente de Insulina" 1996

"Progreso en Inmunología Vol.5, Ámsterdam" 1991-2001

"Standard de Isletas de Anticuerpos de Citoplasma"
 Dibetologia 1986-1993

PharmRCE
Dr. Hugo Romeu M.D.

PHARM RCE

dr.hugoromeu@yahoo.com

PharmRCE

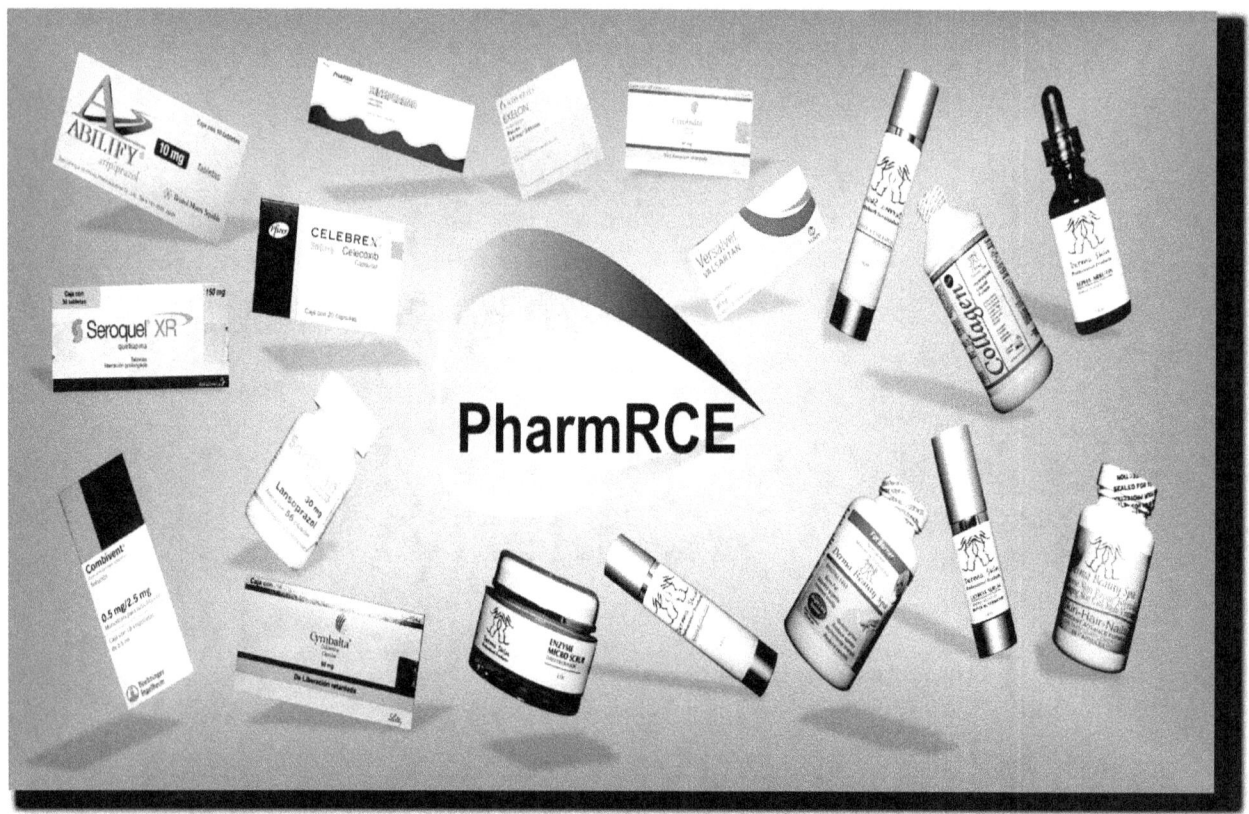

Calle 60 #323A, Colonia Centro, Merida, Tycatan. Mexico 97000
Phone: Cell 1-(305)-627 3703   (999) 287 3142
www.pharmrce.com.mx

PharmRCE es una distribuidora de medicamentos y artículos relacionados con el área de la salud con sede en Mexico.

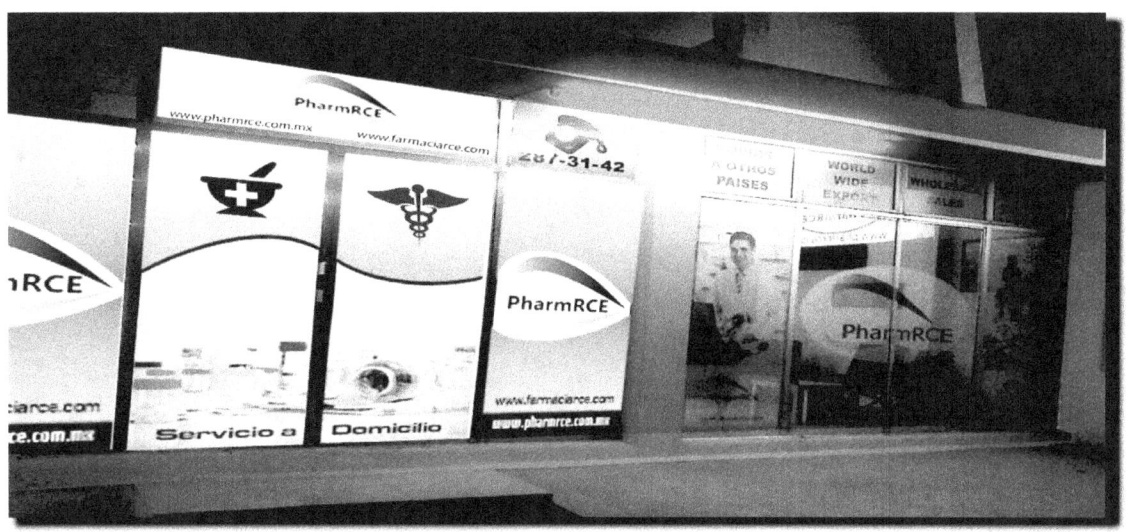

Nuestra operación diaria gira alrededor de nuestros clientes y el objetivo principal de la compañía es garantizar que usted como cliente reciba un servicio impecable , que incluya calidad, cortesía, economía y rapidez , todo esto dentro de una sombrilla de amor y respeto.

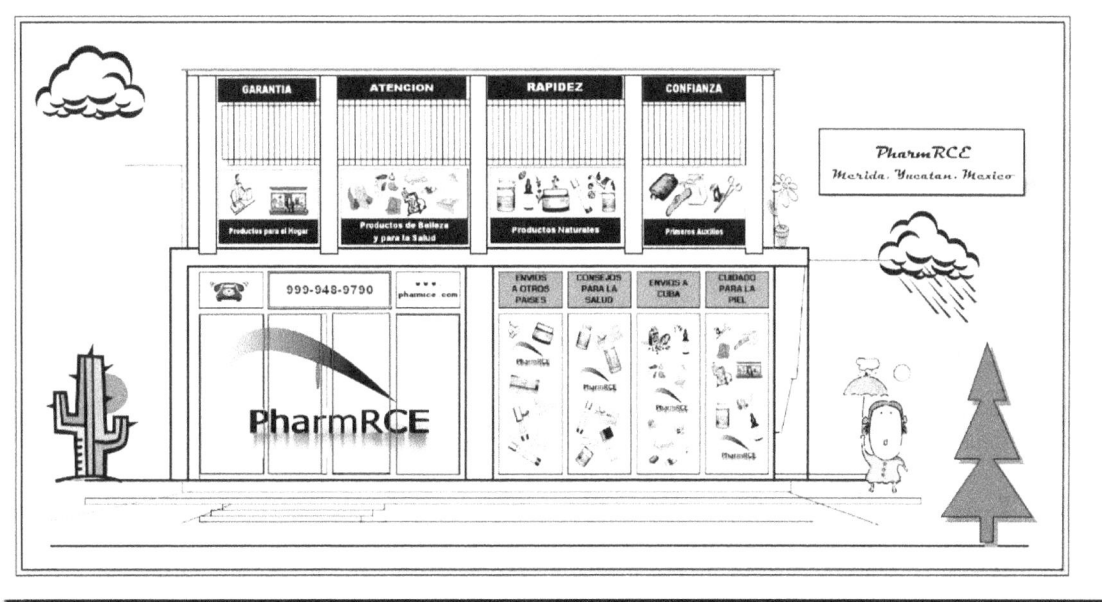

Podemos suministrarle a usted, a sus familiares o a sus amigos cualquier tipo de medicina no controlada, ya sea en su propio domicilio o en el de la persona necesitada en su país de origen, de una manera segura e inmediata.

No somos ajenos a las dificultades que atraviesan los residentes en Mexico para hacerles llegar los muy necesarios medicamentos a sus seres queridos en partes alejadas del pais, ademas en Centro y Sur America y en el Caribe, nuestro propósito es hacer de esa tarea algo agradable y eficaz.

Este por encima de las dificultades, resolver esa necesaria comunicación es uno de los objetivos de PharmRCE , como bien cito el filosofo Nietzche "Todo lo que se hace por amor, se hace mas alla del bien y del mal"

Conviertase en nuestro cliente, haga un primer envio y quedara asombrado con la eficiencia y rapidez con que le brindamos nuestros servicios, hablamos el lenguaje humano , hablamos su idioma, usamos métodos viables y efectivos para que desde la comodidad de su hogar pueda encargar productos para ser entregados donde usted lo requiera, de manera responsable a la persona que usted desee.

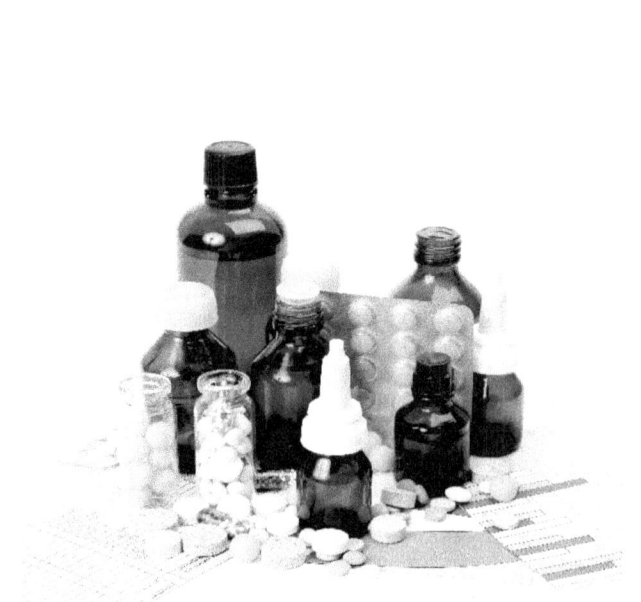

Usando nuestra pagina en el Internet se sentirá cómodo, el hecho de ordenar un producto medicinal no será complejo, sino por el contrario, sea fluido y comprensible y nuestros operadores le atenderán caso de que sea necesario, con eficiencia y paciencia ante cualquier dificultad que presente su orden.

En nuestra pagina web, podrá encontrar las listas con la gama de productos que podemos suministrar o si lo prefiere puede comunicarse con nosotros y le enviaremos las listas de los productos que se ajusten a su necesidad.

*PharmRCE México, ofrece algunos
conjuntos pre diseñados, con el propósito
que de manera fácil se pueda cubrir de
inmediato algunas necesidades básicas específicas.*

Algunos de los "paquetes" disponibles:

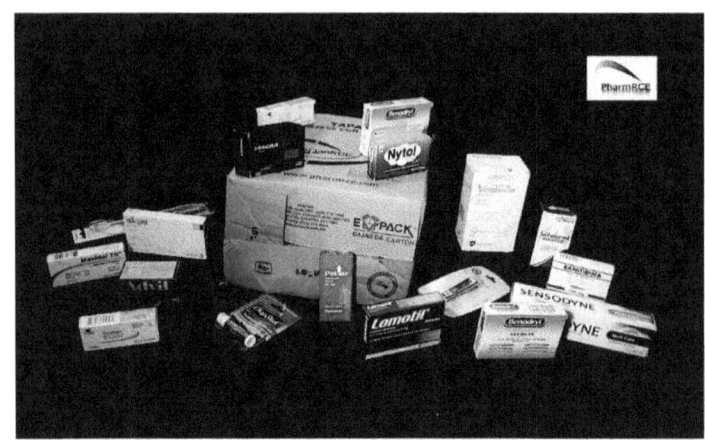

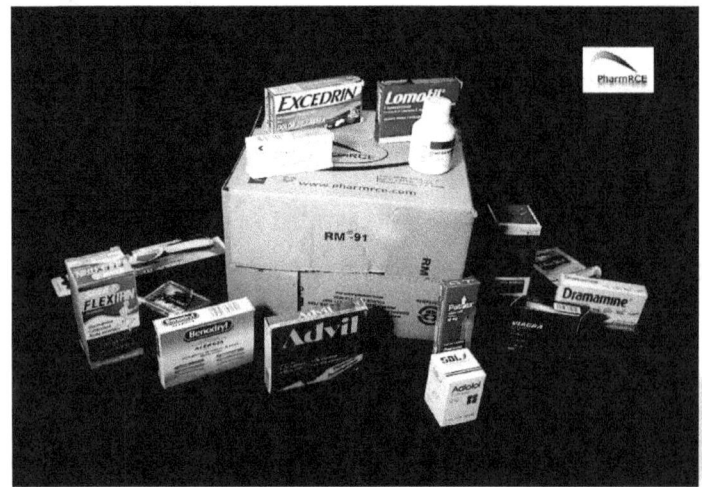

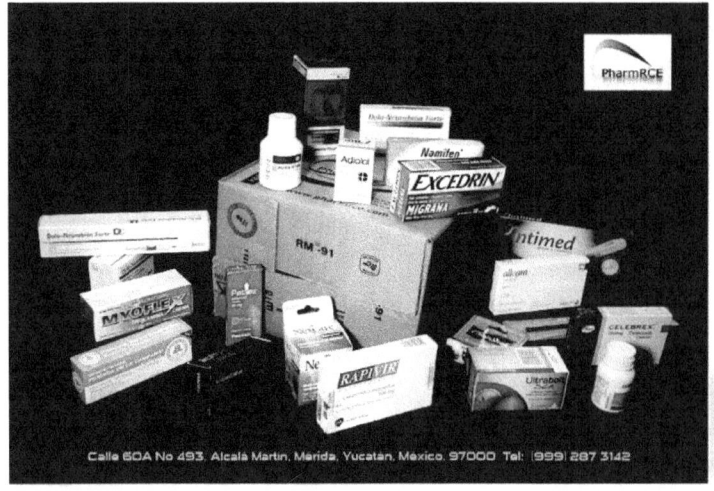

Paquetes (kits)

Según necesidades especificas.

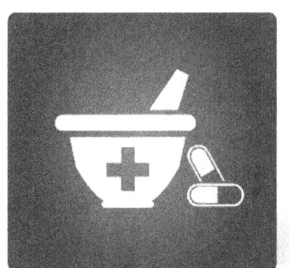

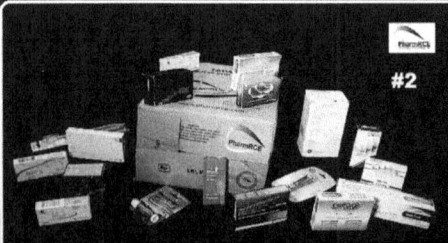

#2

1-APODEFIL SILDENAFIL CAJA 4 TAB.
1-KIT DE VIAJE DE CEPILLOS
1-CALADRYL CLEAR FRASCO 180ML.
1-CHAPSTICK 4,2G HUMECTANTE LABIAL
1-BULLENZA SILDENAFIL 100MG 4 TAB.
1-FREESTYLE OPTIUM 25 TIRAS GLUCOSA
1-METAMIZOL SODICO.CAJA 3 AMPOLLETAS.
1-ACTRON IBUPROFENO 200MG 10CAPS.
1-CEPILLO 47 TUFT SUAVE.
1-PRESONE AMLOPINO CAJA 10 TAB

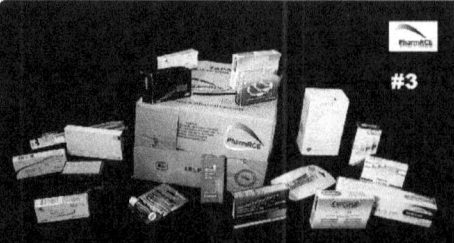

#3

1-CEPILLLO 47 TUFT SUAVE
1-MIBIFON CREMA TUBO 20G.
1-COLGATE SENSITIVE PRO-ALIVIO 35ML.
1-PRO-COLD 666
1-ELITE CALCIO/VITAMINA D3400MG/120UL30TAB.
1-GILLETE FUSION PROGLIDE 198G/200ML
1-TE MANZANILLA 25G 25 SAQUITOS DE 1G.
1-ENI CIPROFLOXACINO 3MG/5ML
1-ACTRON IBUPROFENO 200MG 10CAPS.
1-TUMS 500MG 75 TAB.
1-SPEED STICK 60G.

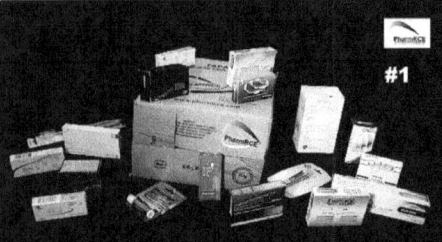

#1

1- ELECTROLIT SUERO 625ML
1- HIPOGLOS CREMA 110G
1- BULLENZA SILDENAFIL 100MG 1 TAB.
1- CINAZEL CARBAMAZEPINA 200MG.20TAB.
1- CRONOCAPS.3MG CAJA 30 CAPS.
1- METAMIZOL SODICO.CAJA 3 AMPOLLETAS.
1- LIPIKAR SURGRAS JABON 80 G.
1- REDOXON 1G.CAJA CON 10 TAB.
1- CEPILLO 47 TUFT MEDIANO.

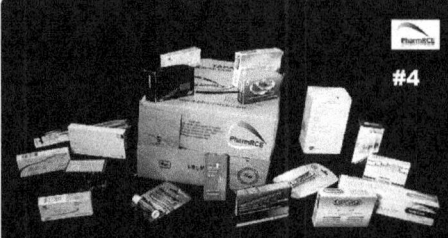

#4

1-DRAMAMINE INFANTIL 25MG 4 SUPOSITORIOS.
1-CALADRYL CALAMINA FRASCO 180ML.
1-MIBIFON CREMA TUBO 20G
1-COLGATE SENSITIVE PRO-ALIVIO 50 G.
1-CINAZEL CARBAMAZEPINA 200MG.20 TAB.
1-CEPILLO 47 TUFT MEDIANO.
1-CHAPSTICK 4,2G HUMECTANTE LABIAL FRESA
1-ACEITE MENNEN 200ML
1-JOHNSONZ BABY JABON 75
1-TALCO MENNEN 100G.ROSA
1-IMALETMETFORMINA-GLIBENCLAMIDA 60 TAB
1-LADY GRECIAN 120ML

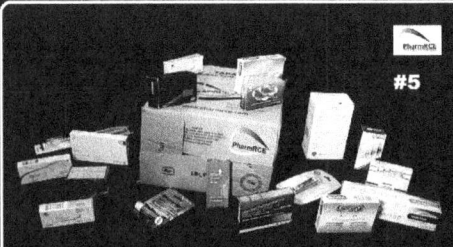

#5

1-TALCO MENNEN 100G.ROSA

1-PRO-COLD 666 24 TAB.

1-COLGATE SENSITIVE PRO.ALIVIO 50G.

1-ELECTROLIT SUERO 625ML

1-CEPILLO47 TUFT MEDIANO

1-LIPIKAR SURGRAS JABON 80 G.

1-JOHNSONZ BABY JABON 75

1-CHAPSTICK4,2G HUMECTANTE LABIAL FRESA

1-GILLETE FUSION PROGLIDE 198G/200ML

1-SPEED STICK 60G.

1-GLUCO VANCE 500MG/2.5MG CAJA 60 TAB.

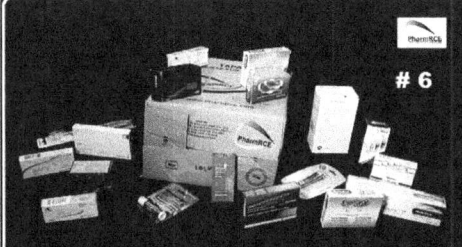

 # 6

1- PONDS CLARANTB3 400ML

1- EXFOLIALING PAPAYA 4FL OZ

1- ULTROX CREAM 1.7 OZ

1- HYALURONIC CREAM 1.7OZ

1- CAVIAR COLLAGEN CREMA 30ML

1- LIPIKAR SURGRAS 80G

1- HINDS HIDRATACION ESENCIAL 230ML

1- MENNEN JABON BABY 110G.

1- ALERGIBON JABON SIN AROMA 120G

1- EXFOLIANTE JABON 100g

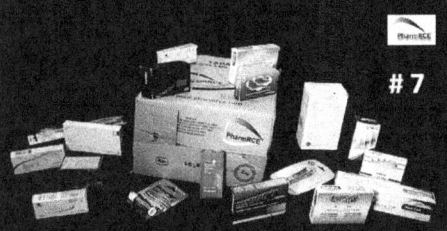

 # 7

1- VITACILINA ESENCIAL JABON 100g

1- ENZYME MICRO SCRUB 1 OZ

1- VITAMINA E Y ALOE VERA

1- GREEN TEA SPF30+ 1.7 OZ

1- ALERGIBON JABON SIN AROMA120G

1- LIPIKAR SURGRAS 80G

1- HINDS HIDRATACION ESENCIAL 230ML

1- PONDS CLARANTB3 200ML

1- MENNEN JABON BABY 110G.

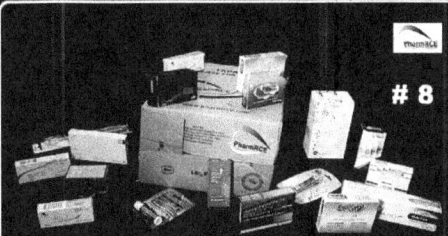

 # 8

1- APODEFIL SILDENAFIL 100MG CON 1 TAB.

1- EURODERM CLOTRIMAZOL 2% CREMA

1- BENADRYL CAJA 24 TAB.

1- 20 ADVIL IBUPROFENO 200 mg

1- DRAMAMINE DIMENHIDRINATO 50 mg 24 TAB.

1- THOROMBOCID FORTE CREMA FACIAL60 G.

1- INSUCAR DINITRATO DE 10 mg

1- ULTROX CREAM 1.7 OZ

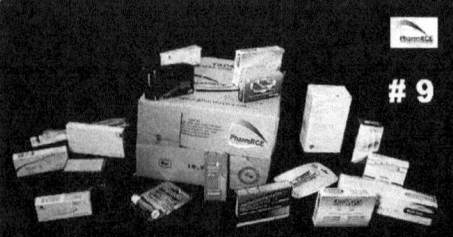

 # 9

1- LUBRIDERM PIEL NORMAL
   240ML.
1- RANITIDINA 150mg caja
   20 TAB.
1- 1 TAB. SILDENAFIL 50mg
1- 14 PREGABALINA 75 mg
1- SENSODYNE CREMA 113g
1- LOPRESOR*R 20 TAB.
   METOPROLOL 95mg
1- CEPILLO ORBIT MEDIANO

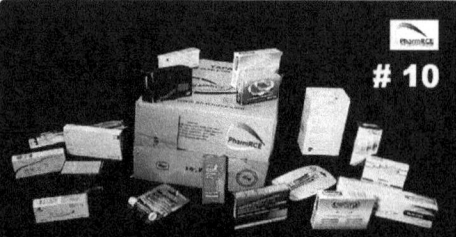

 # 10

1- ASEPXIA GEL 28g
1- SILDENAFIL 50mg caja 4 TAB.
1- RANITIDINA 150mg 20 TAB.
1- PREGABALINA 150 mg 28 caps.
1- LOPRESOR*R METOPROLOL
   95mg 20 tab.
1- CEPILLO 47 TUFT MEDIANO
1- SPEED STICK 48HORAS
1- TALCO O-DOLEX 150g
   NATURALS

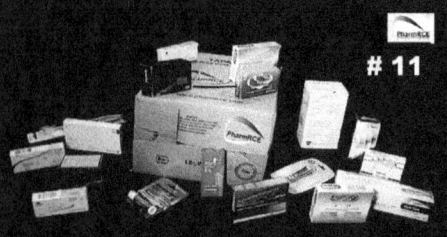

 # 11

1- EXFOLIANTE JABON 100g
1- NAMIFEN Acido mefenamico
   500mg 20 TAB.
1- 10 T ADVIL IBUPROFENO 200MG
1- LEVONORGESTREL 0.75 mg 2 T
1- ESKAPAR 400mg caja 16 CAPS.
1- BIOMETRIX FRASCO 30 CAPS.
1- DRAMAMINE DIMENHIDRINATO
   25 mg 4 susp.
1- BENADRYL CAJA 24 TAB.
1- EURODERM CLOTRIMAZOL
   CREMA 2%
1- DERMAN CREMA 50g.

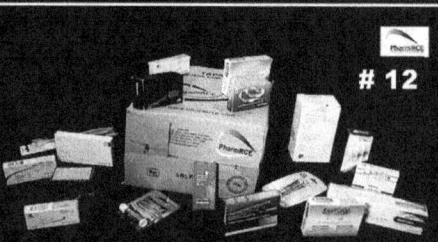

 # 12

1- AMOXICILINA 500MG 12 CAPS.
1- DALATINA-V* CLIDAMICINA
   2% CREMA
1- MIBIFON BIFONAZOL
   CREMA 20G.
1- METAMIZOL SODICO C 3 Amp
1- INSUSYM GLIBENCLAMIDA 5mg
   50TAB.
1- ALOPURINOL 300mg 30TAB.
1- ACICLOVIR CREMA 5%
1- 28 T ARIZIC TOPIRAMATO
1- 10 ADVIL IBUPROFENO 200MG
1- ENSURE SABOR VAINILLA 400

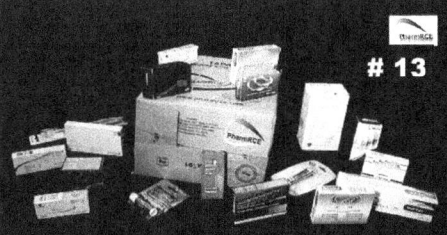

 # 13

1- GILLETTE FUSION 198g/200ml
1- ENSURE SABOR FRESA 400
1- ACOMEXOL CREMA 30g.
1- VITACILINA ESC. JABON 100 g
1- BALSAMO CASTRO SPORT
   FRASCO 50ML.
1- ENAPRIL 10mg CON 30 TAB.
1- MIBIFON BIFONAZOL CREM 20G.
1- AMOXICILINA 500MG 12 CAPS.
1- DALATINA-V* CLIDAMICINA 2%
   CREMA
1- IRBESARTAN 300mg 28 TAB

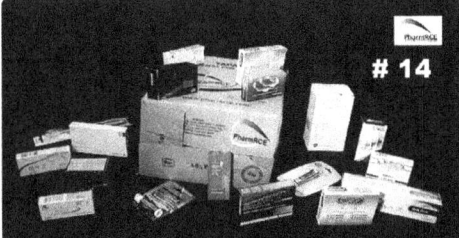

 # 14

1- ELECTROLIT SUERO 625ML
1- MIBIFON CREMA 20G
1- HIPOGLOS CREMA 110G
1- JABON EXFOLIANTE 100G
1- RANITIDINA 20 TAB.150MG
1- ADVIL IBUPROFENO200MG
   CON 10 CAPS.
1- CELL-VITAL GO CON 60 CAPS.
1- ARRETIN ACIDO RETINOICO
   0.05%TUBO30G.
1- HINDS CLASICA 90ML.
1- ILIADIN AGUA NASAL30ML.

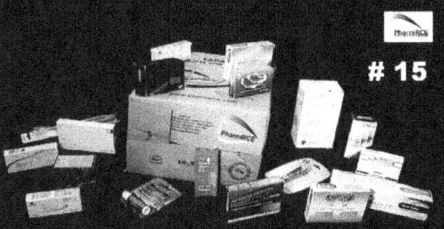

 # 15

1- ELECTROLIT SUERO 625ML
1- ARRETIN ACIDO RETINOICO
   0.05%TUBO30G.
1- CELL-VITAL GO CON 60 CAPS.
1- ADVIL IBUPROFENO 200MG10 C.
1- JABON EXFOLIANTE 100G
1- HINDS NATURAL 90ML.
1- CEPILLO47TUFT SUAVE
1- DIVADAYS 550MG 12 TAB.
1- PRO;COLD666 24 TAB.
1- DRAMAMINE JARABE INFANTIL
   120ML

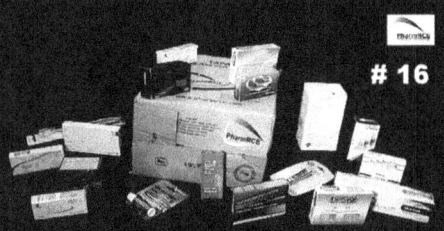

 # 16

1- ELECTROLIT SUERO 625ML
1- JABON EXFOLIANTE 100G
1- ADVIL IBUPROFENO200MG
   CON 10 CAPS.
1- RANITIDINA 20 TAB.150MG
1- CEPILLO SMART GRIP MADIANO
1- ELITE AMOXICILINA 500MG
   CON 12 CAPS.
1- SIMIPAZ FORTE 30CAPS.
1- SAMONIL-V 500MG CON 10 TAB.
1- HIDROCORTISONA CREMA
   1MG TUBO 15G.

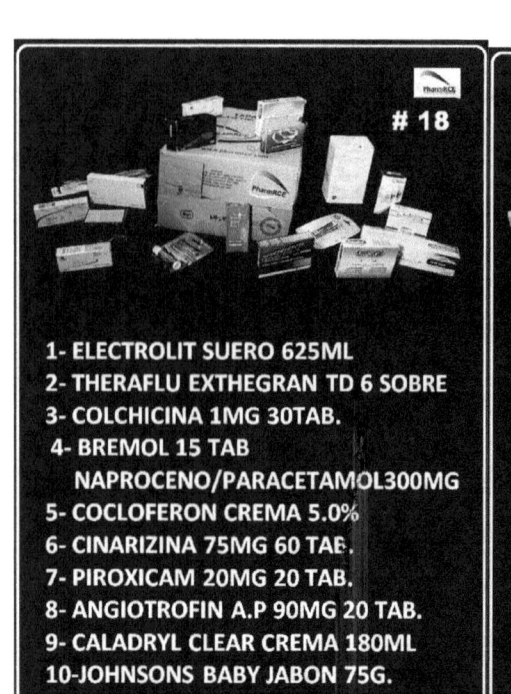

 # 18

1- ELECTROLIT SUERO 625ML
2- THERAFLU EXTHEGRAN TD 6 SOBRE
3- COLCHICINA 1MG 30TAB.
 4- BREMOL 15 TAB
    NAPROCENO/PARACETAMOL300MG
5- COCLOFERON CREMA 5.0%
6- CINARIZINA 75MG 60 TAB.
7- PIROXICAM 20MG 20 TAB.
8- ANGIOTROFIN A.P 90MG 20 TAB.
9- CALADRYL CLEAR CREMA 180ML
10-JOHNSONS BABY JABON 75G.

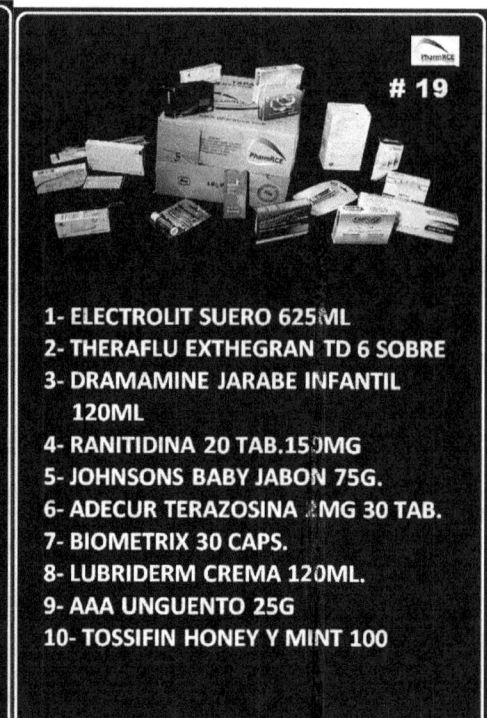

 # 19

1- ELECTROLIT SUERO 625ML
2- THERAFLU EXTHEGRAN TD 6 SOBRE
3- DRAMAMINE JARABE INFANTIL
   120ML
4- RANITIDINA 20 TAB.150MG
5- JOHNSONS BABY JABON 75G.
6- ADECUR TERAZOSINA 2MG 30 TAB.
7- BIOMETRIX 30 CAPS.
8- LUBRIDERM CREMA 120ML.
9- AAA UNGUENTO 25G
10- TOSSIFIN HONEY Y MINT 100

Como citó el escritor norteamericano Ralph Emerson

"La primera riqueza es la salud"

y usted y su familia merecen tener a su alcance medicina de primer orden.

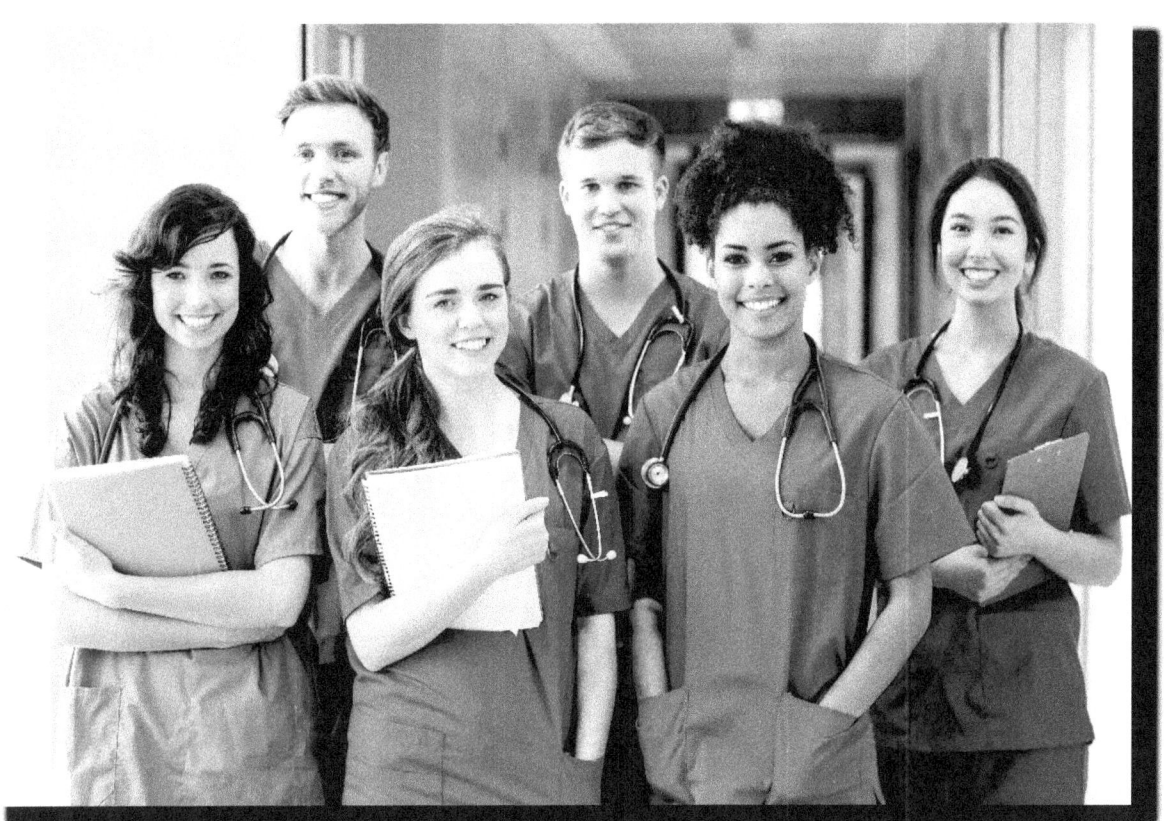

Responda a las necesidades medicinales de su familia de una manera discreta y fluida usando los servicios de PharmRCE.

PharmRCE es una farmacia en línea, creada para usted.
Con clientes alrededor del mundo, que están satisfechos a la repuesta inmediata de las necesidades medicinales de su familia de una manera discreta y sin costuras, usar PharmRCE.

Según Diagnósticos.

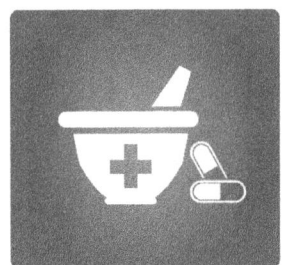

Antibiotics

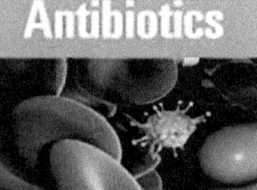

Antidepresivos

Anti-Hongos

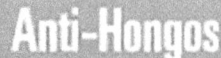

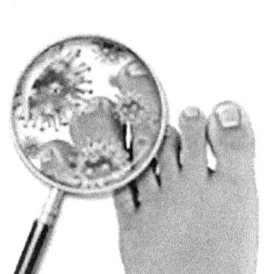

Asma

Anticonceptivos

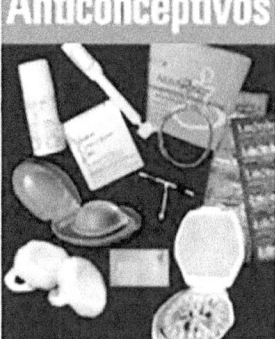

Presion Sanguinea

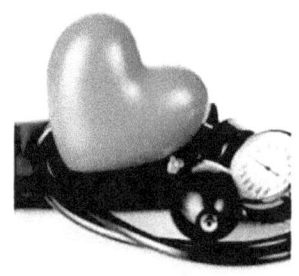

Cirrosis

Diabetes

Desinfectante

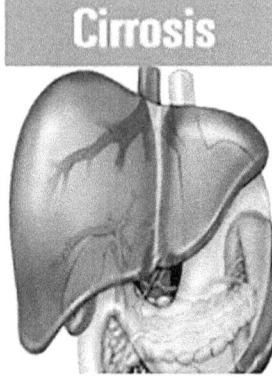

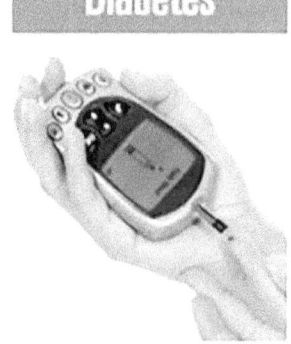

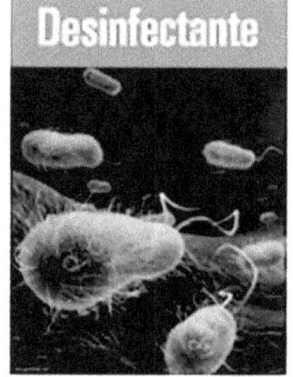

Sida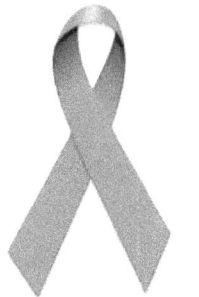

Alergias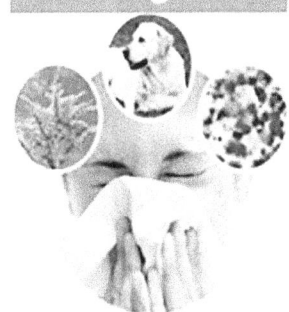

Antibacterial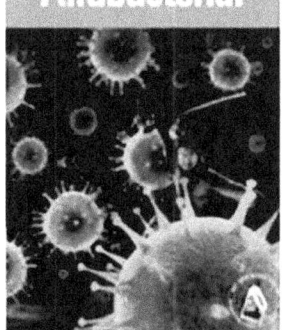

Antiinflamatorio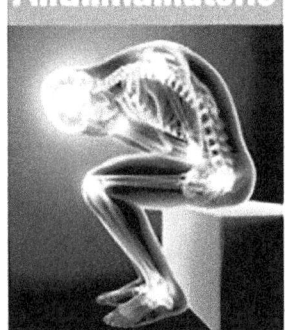

Anti-viral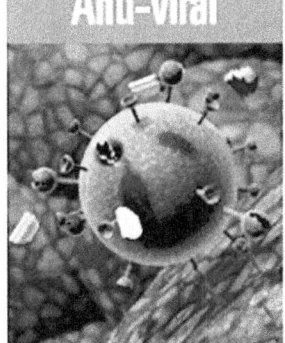

Artritis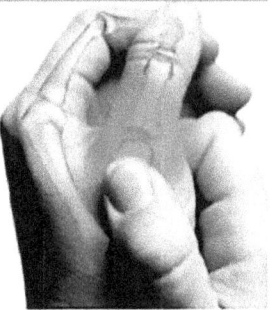

Cancer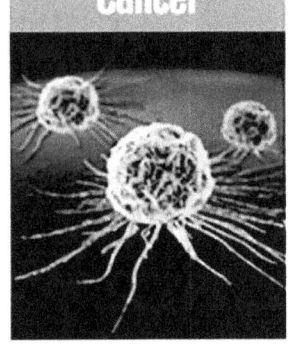

Cardiovascular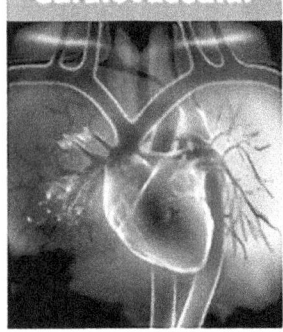

Colesterol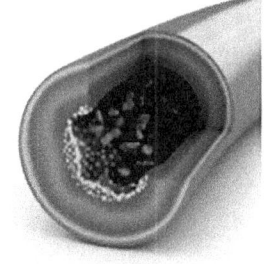

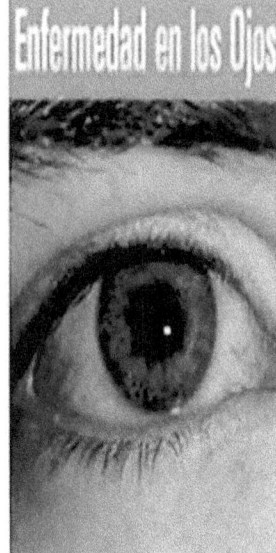

Enfermedad en los Ojos

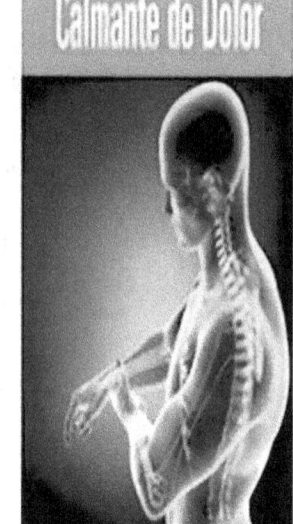

Calmante de Dolor

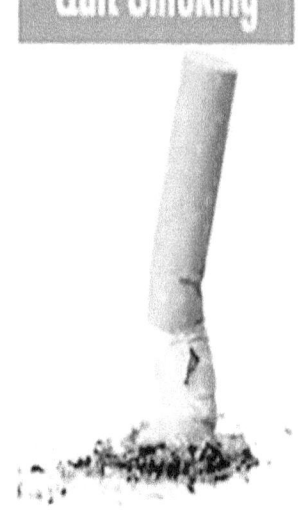

Quit Smoking

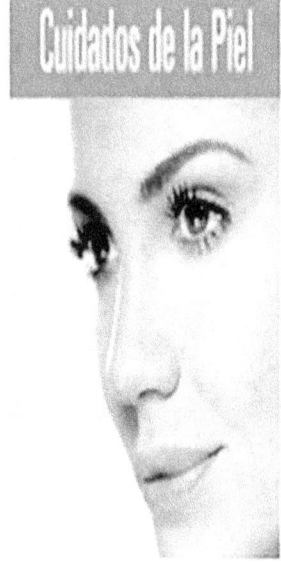

Cuidados de la Piel

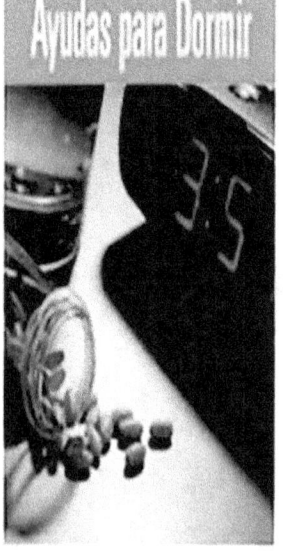

Ayudas para Dormir

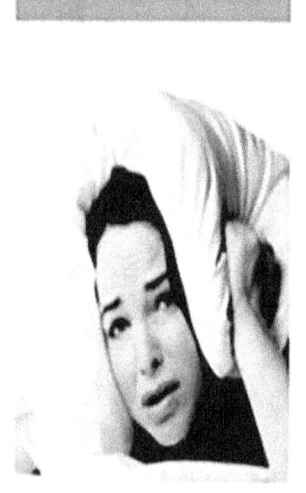

Transtornos del Sueño

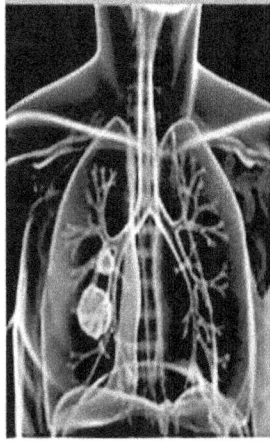

Respiratory Disease

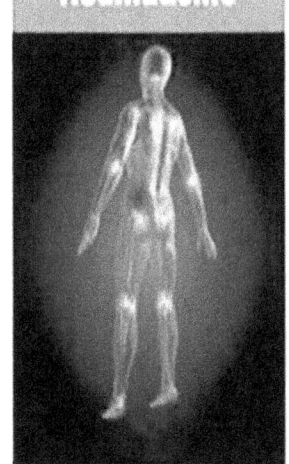

Reumatismo

Enfermedades Sexuales

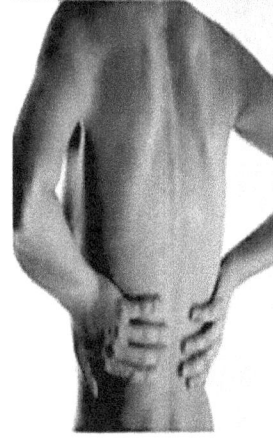

ACIDO URICO

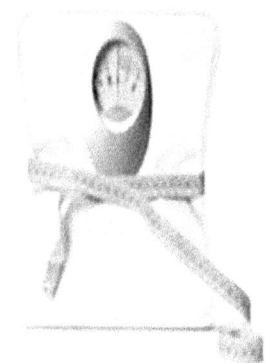

Perdida de Peso

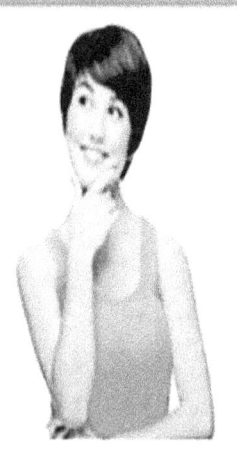

Salud Femenina

Diuretico

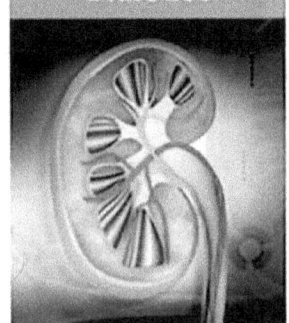

Disfuncion Erectil

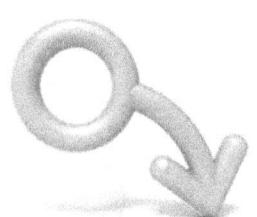

Gotas para Ojos

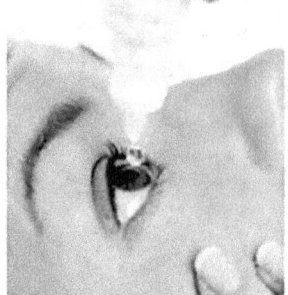

Perdida de Cabello

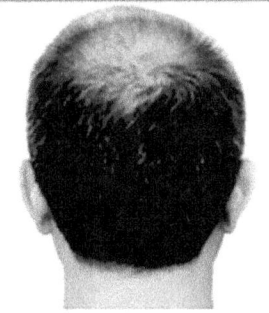

Hemorroides

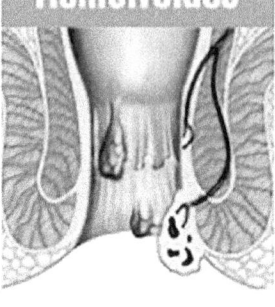

Hepatitis C

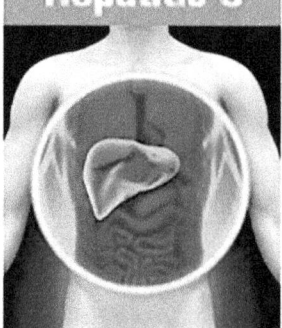

Enfermedad en Riñones

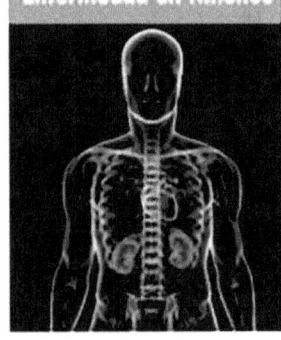

Salud Para el Hombre

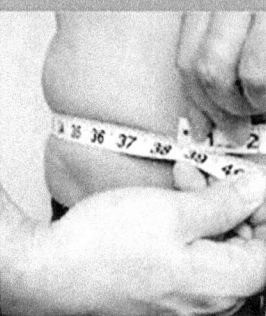

Paquete para hombres

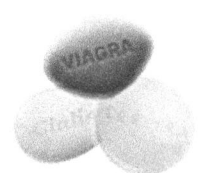

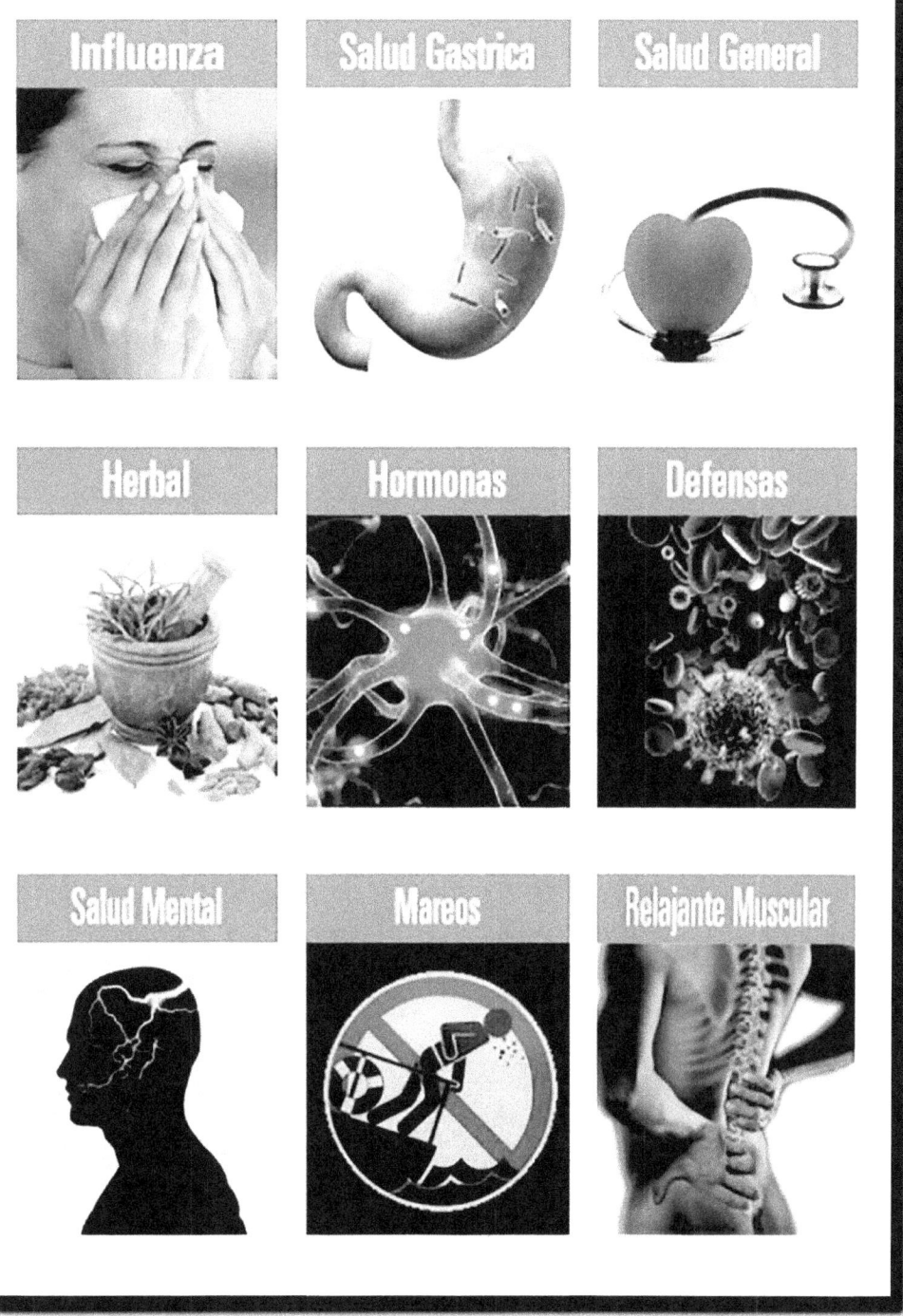

Con el uso de nuestra página web, usted se sentirá cómodo. Solicitar un medicamento no es difícil, pero por el contrario, es una tarea muy sencilla que nuestros operadores están dispuestos a completar por usted.

www.farmaciarce.com.mx

PharmRCE, tiene una Empresa hermana en los Estados Unidos,

PharmRCE USA, localizada en el estado de Georgia:

PharmRCE USA

**2201 Osborne Road, Saint Marys, Camdem County
Georgia 31558**

1-(912) 510 4900

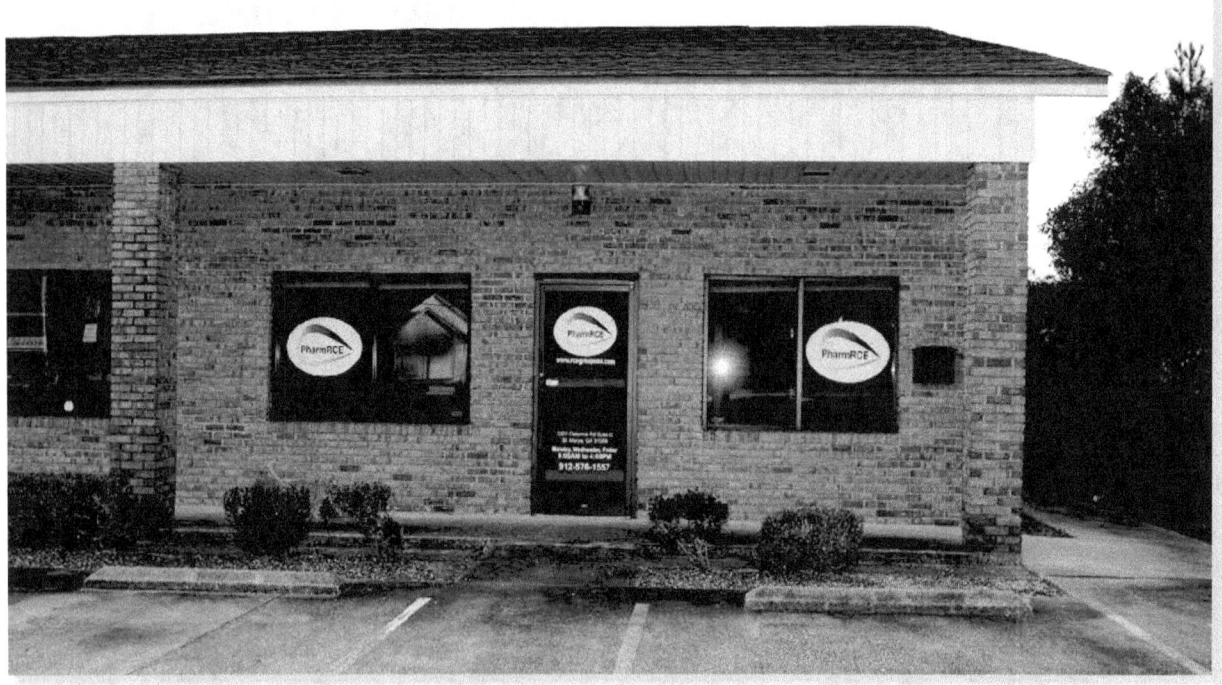

Pharmrce México, AKA FarmaciaRCE,
es parte de RCE Group USA,
que radica en los Estados Unidos.

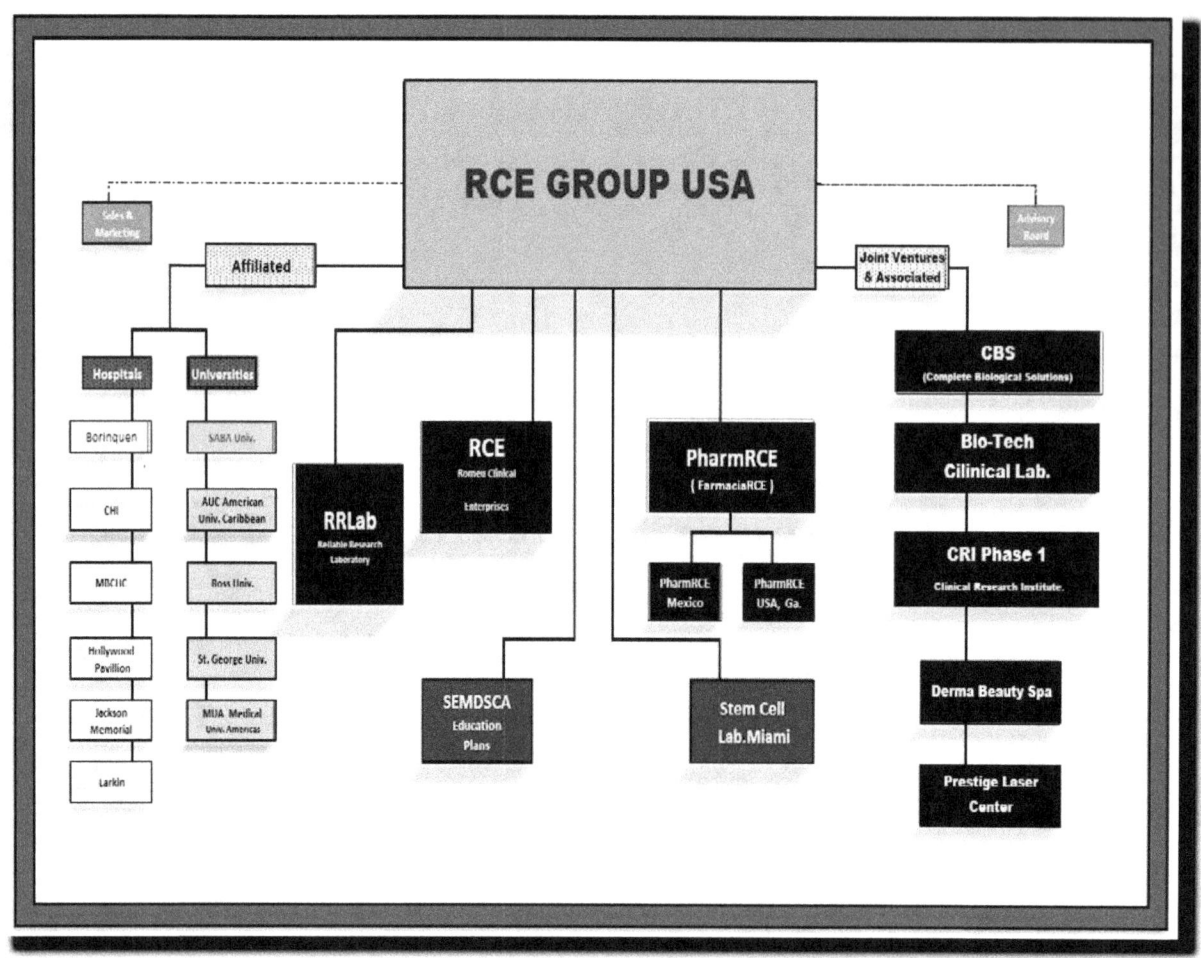

ORGANIGRAMA RCE GROUP USA

Reliable Research Laboratory
Dr. Hugo Romeu M.D.

RELIABLE RESEARCH
LABORATORY

dr.hugoromeu@yahoo.com

Reliable Research Laboratory

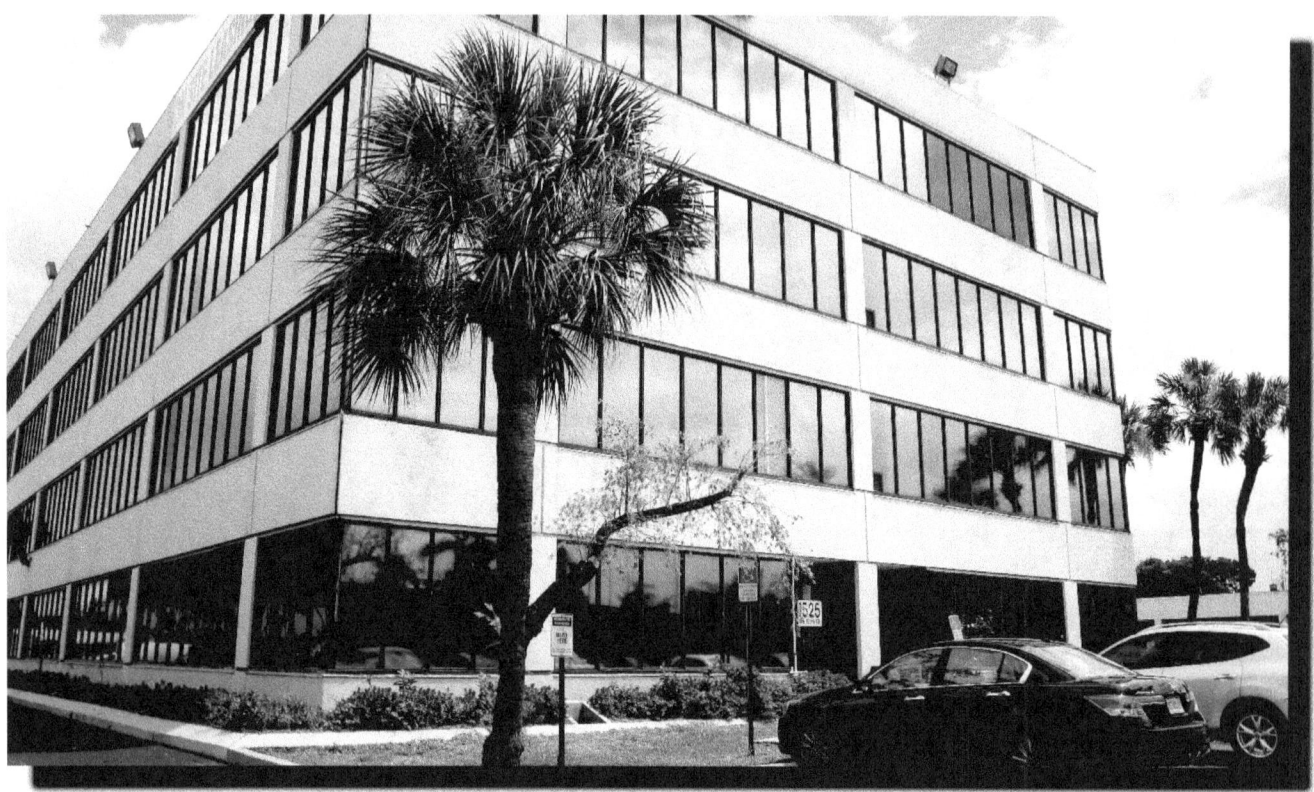

1525 NW 167 St Suite. Miami Gardens, Fl 33169
Phone: (305) 627 3703 Fax: (786) 916 3296
www.reliableresearchlaboratory.com

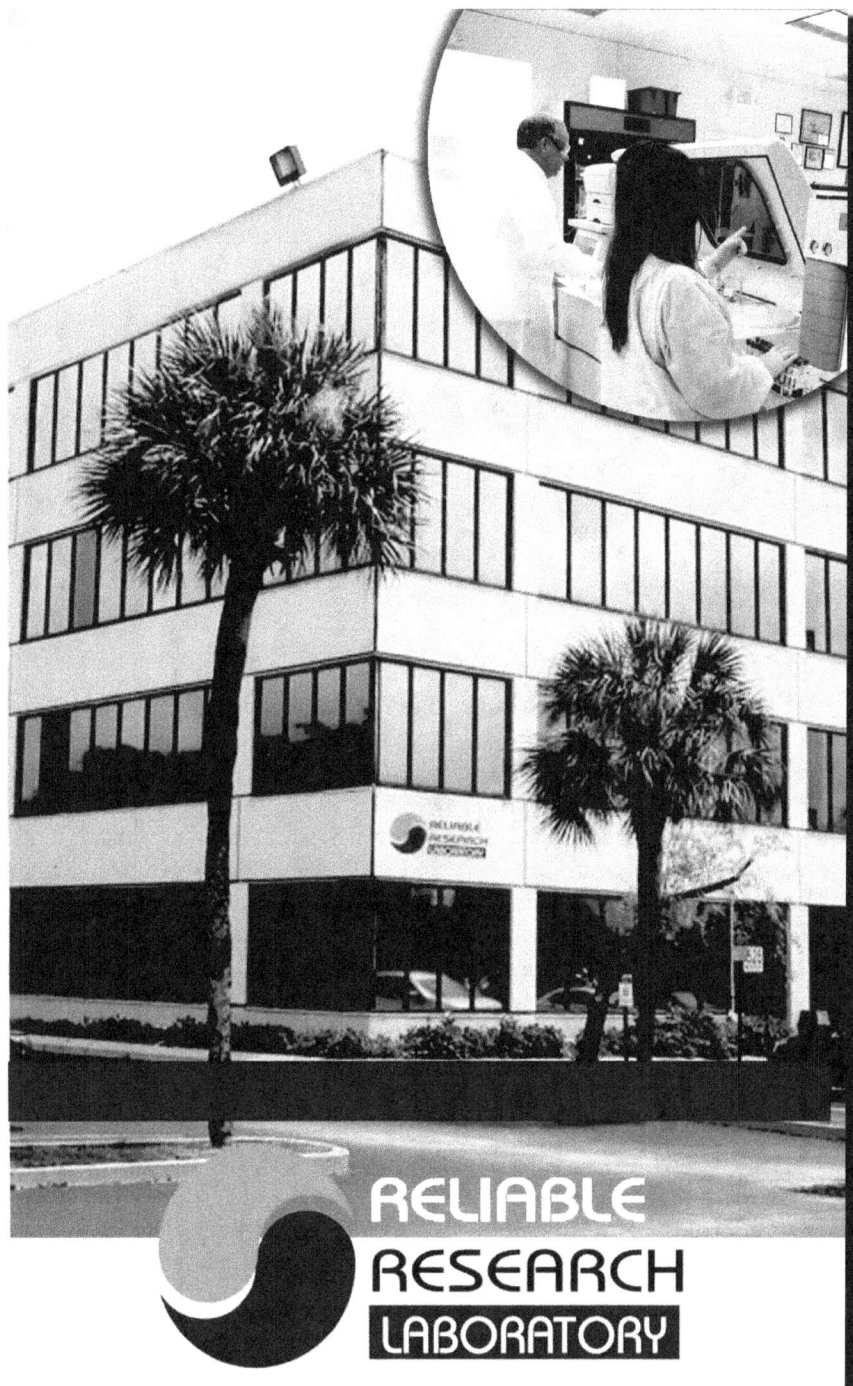

RELIABLE
RESEARCH
LABORATORY

Fast and reliable results

📞 305-625-2183

www.rerelab.com
www.reliableresearchlaboratory.com

Reliable Research Laboratory is a full service Clinical Laboratory which is licensed and equipped to perform testing in all areas of medicine. We are certified by CLIA,COLA,AHCA and CAP.

Our team has been together for over 22 years, and we have the equipment, training and experience to complete the task of reliable and reproducible lab data.

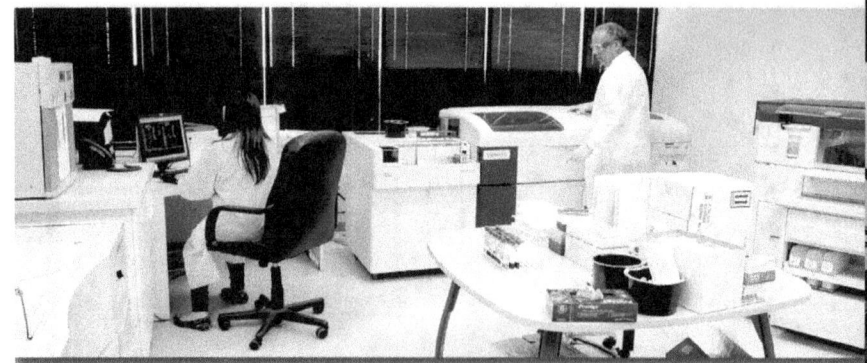

The completion of over 1600 Clinical trial studies has given us the stand alone reputation of simply the best in the research arena.

RRL is your partner in any task. We not only perform the actual lab testing; our experts will assist in every facet from compliance to regulatory affairs.

The principal owner, Hugo Romeu, MD is a pathologist with over 32 years of experience in Laboratory Medicine, with a special interest in compound development, and clinical correlation of the lab data.

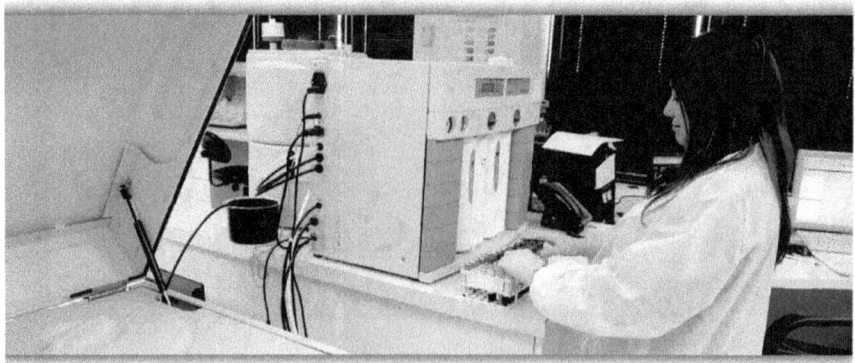

Our staff is complete with one of the most qualified and renowned laboratory specialist's, John Shultz. He was trained at John Hopkins and has been managing and directing laboratories for over 25 years.

Every member of our team has been hand-picked to deliver accurate and reliable results.

If you're looking for state of the art technology, speed and accuracy ,RRL is the lab for you

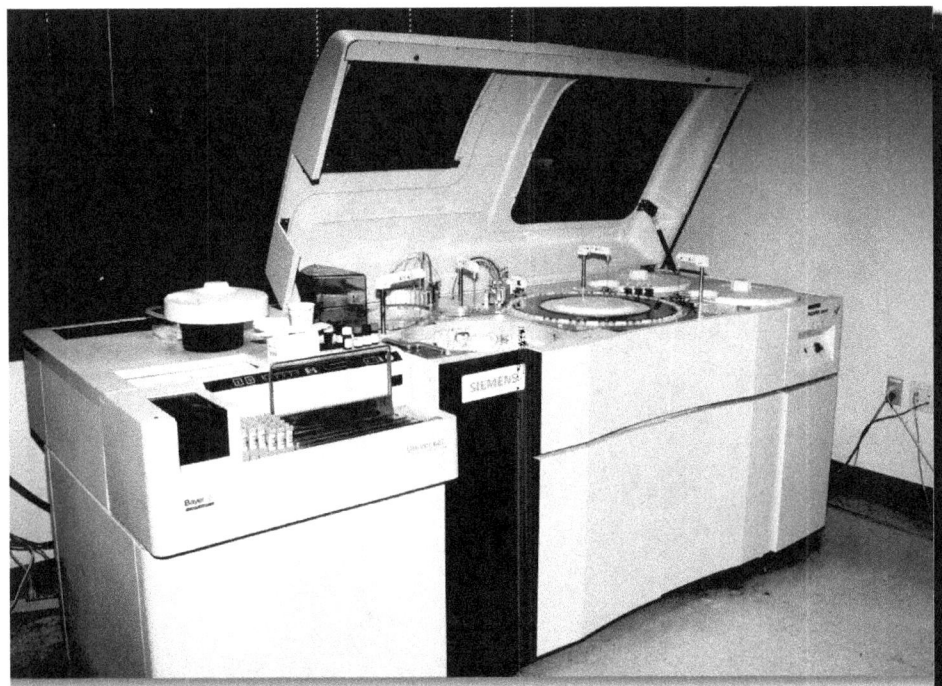

A laboratory is only as good as its personnel and equipment. Everything starts at the top and reflected in the entire staff and infrastructure. Dr. Romeu and John Shultz have been trained in the most prestigious institutions; which include Roswell Park Memorial Institute, SUNY, Cook County Hospital, John Hopkins. They have been working together for over 25 years directing and managing some of the largest clinical laboratories in the State of Florida. Dr. Romeu has served in government positions as a Medical Examiner and expert in toxicology and APCP, in addition to being the Chief of Pathology in several hospitals and Laboratories. John has been running complex clinical laboratories with a hands on approach in technical and administrative management. The second tier of the leadership team has been working with senior management for over 18 years. We invite you to join our family of reliable experts in laboratory medicine.

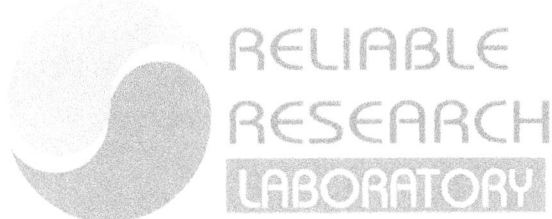

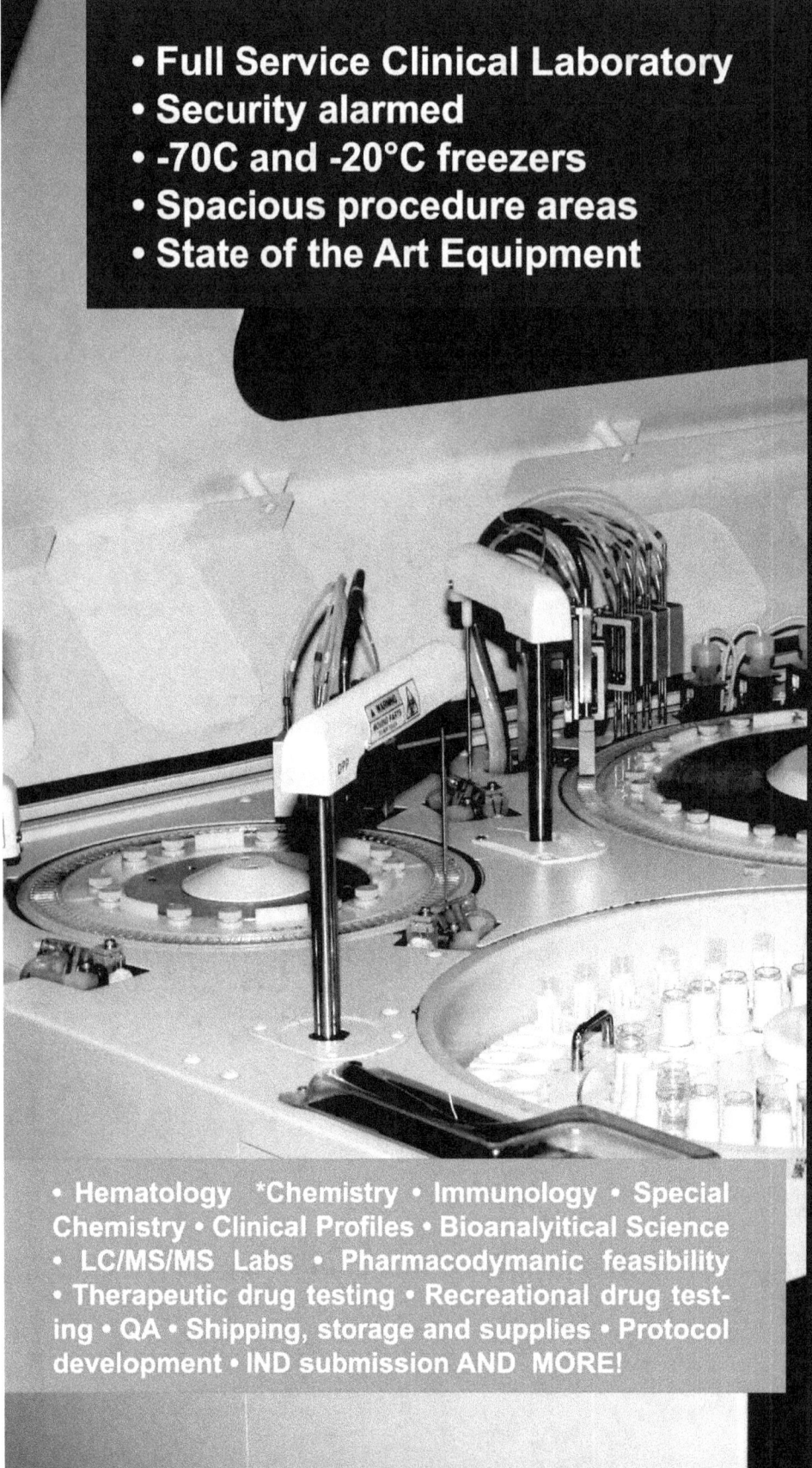

- Full Service Clinical Laboratory
- Security alarmed
- -70C and -20°C freezers
- Spacious procedure areas
- State of the Art Equipment

• Hematology *Chemistry • Immunology • Special Chemistry • Clinical Profiles • Bioanalyitical Science • LC/MS/MS Labs • Pharmacodymanic feasibility • Therapeutic drug testing • Recreational drug testing • QA • Shipping, storage and supplies • Protocol development • IND submission AND MORE!

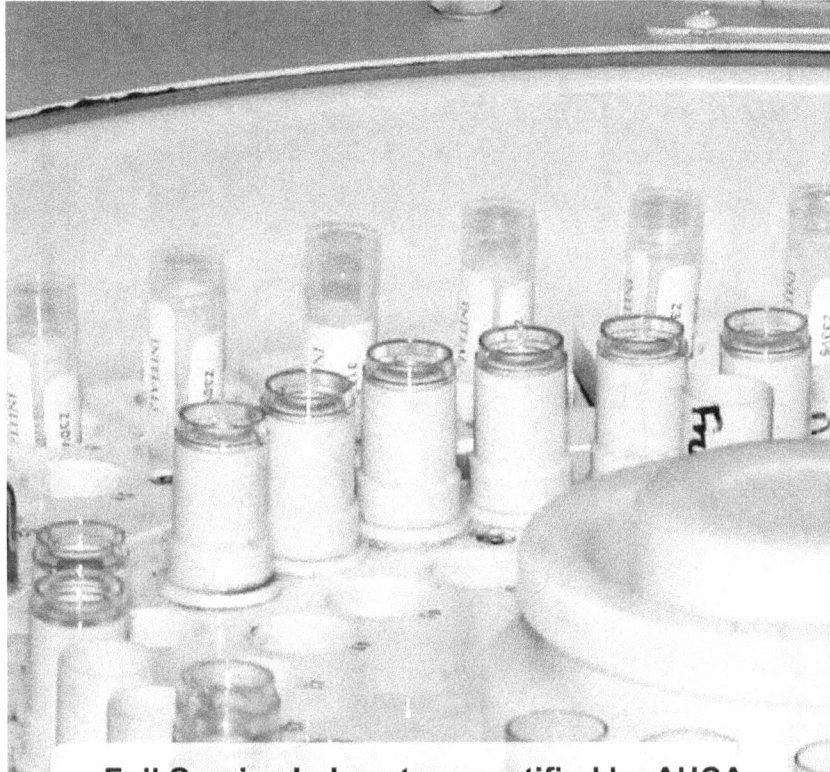

RELIABLE RESEARCH LABORATORY

- **Full Service Laboratory, certified by AHCA, COLA, CLIA, CAP . 99% of our testing is performed in house.**
- **Protocol development. Personalized design of lab manuals, assistance with inclusion and exclusion criteria, visit specific requisitions,**
- **Secure Worldwide internet access to real time laboratory data. Our Laboratory Information Systems are certified, 21 CFR part 11 Compliant & Validated.**
- **Electronic Data Transfers with generic or customized formatting. RRL Delivers data, Quickly and Accurately.**
- **Individualized custom profiles complete with Kit manufacturing, labeling, specimen handling and processing, sample tracking, expedited shipping and turnaround.**
- **Storage, freezers. Secure and safe with alarm systems.**
- **Project Management, On site Pathologist and full time technical staff.**

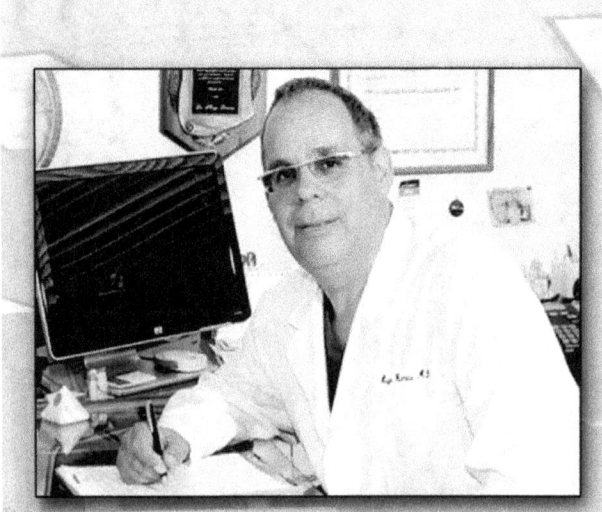

We invite you to discover the ways in which our innovative approaches can cut completion time in half for key types of studies, as well as learn about our customized approaches to serving large pharma, small to mid-size biopharma and generic drug companies – approaches that have made us the industry's leading Central Laboratory.

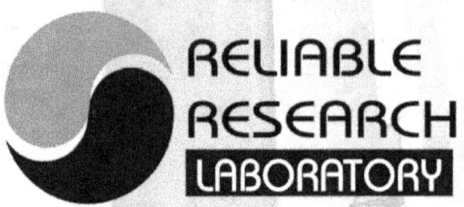

RELIABLE RESEARCH LABORATORY

305-625-2183

www.rerelab.com
www.reliableresearchlaboratory.com
info@rerelab.com

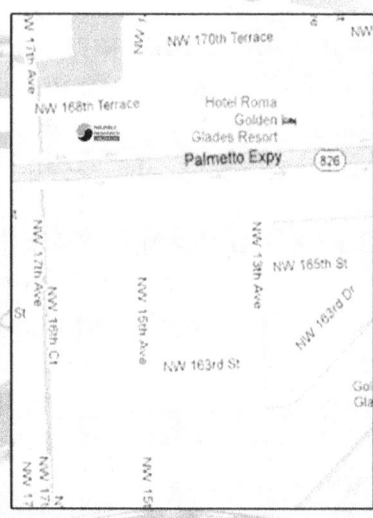

1525 NW 167 St. Suite 140
Miami Gardens, FL, 33169
Fax 305- 625-7106

Reliable Research Laboratory is a pharmaceutical research Clinical Laboratory with the infrastructure and personnel to complete the arduous task of reliable and reproducible scientific research. The core participants in our leadership team have been working together

Reliable Research Laboratory is a pharmaceutical research Clinical Laboratory with the infrastructure and personnel to complete the arduous task of reliable and reproducible scientific research. The core participants in our leadership team have been working together for over 22 years. Together we have completed over 700 studies for all the major global pharmaceutical companies. Our staff of clinicians, pathologists,

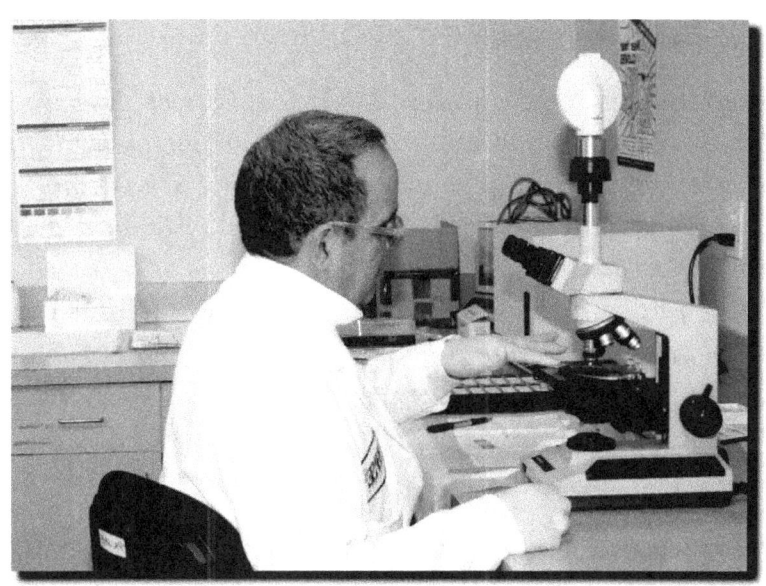

technologists, is complimented with an in house legal team to oversee the regulatory affairs and any compliance issue.

Principal owner of Reliable Research Lab is a Pathologist with 32 years of research experience, with direct involvement in every phase of compound development. From pre-clinical trials, protocol and laboratory design to front line investigator work. The entire team was handpicked for their life time of contributions to the research

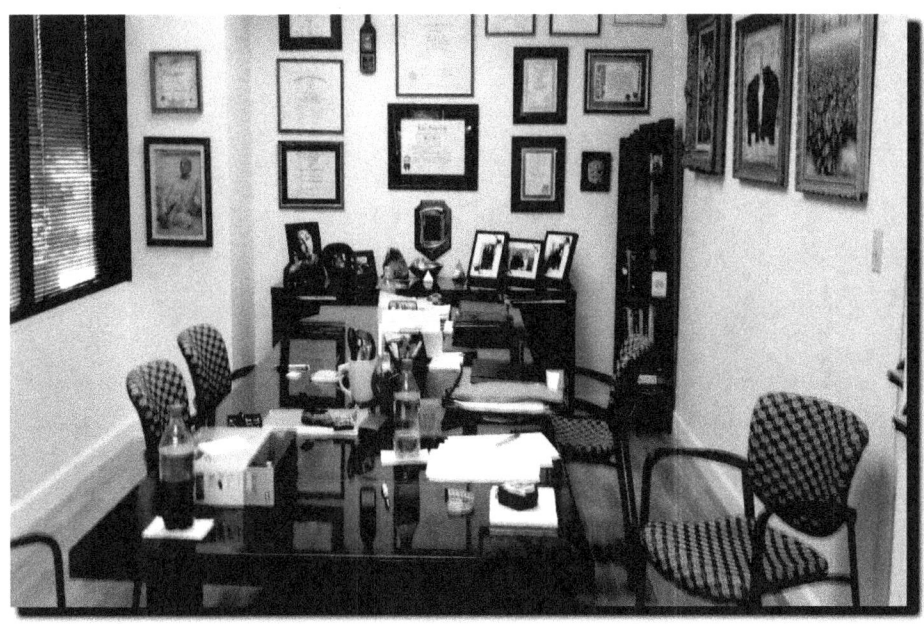

industry. Every single member of our staff has been involved in hundreds of complex studies of all phases. We take pride in our practical and proven experience in the development and establishment of safe medicines which have revolutionized the treatment of the most common afflictions.

Reliable Research Lab is a viable option for any pharmaceutical company because of the infrastructure, extensive training and practical experience of the entire staff. There are key individuals in leadership roles to oversee the entire operation. Take the time to read about our team

Hugo Romeu, M.D. Chief Executive Officer Executive Medical Director Dr. Hugo Romeu received formal training in experimental laboratory medicine at several prestigious institutions such as Roswell Park Memorial Institute, State University of New York and Cook County Hospital. He has published, written protocols and participated in study designs in all phases of research, from pre-clinical animal trials to late phase studies. Over the last 32 years he has completed 672 trials, the majority phase one and bioequivalence.

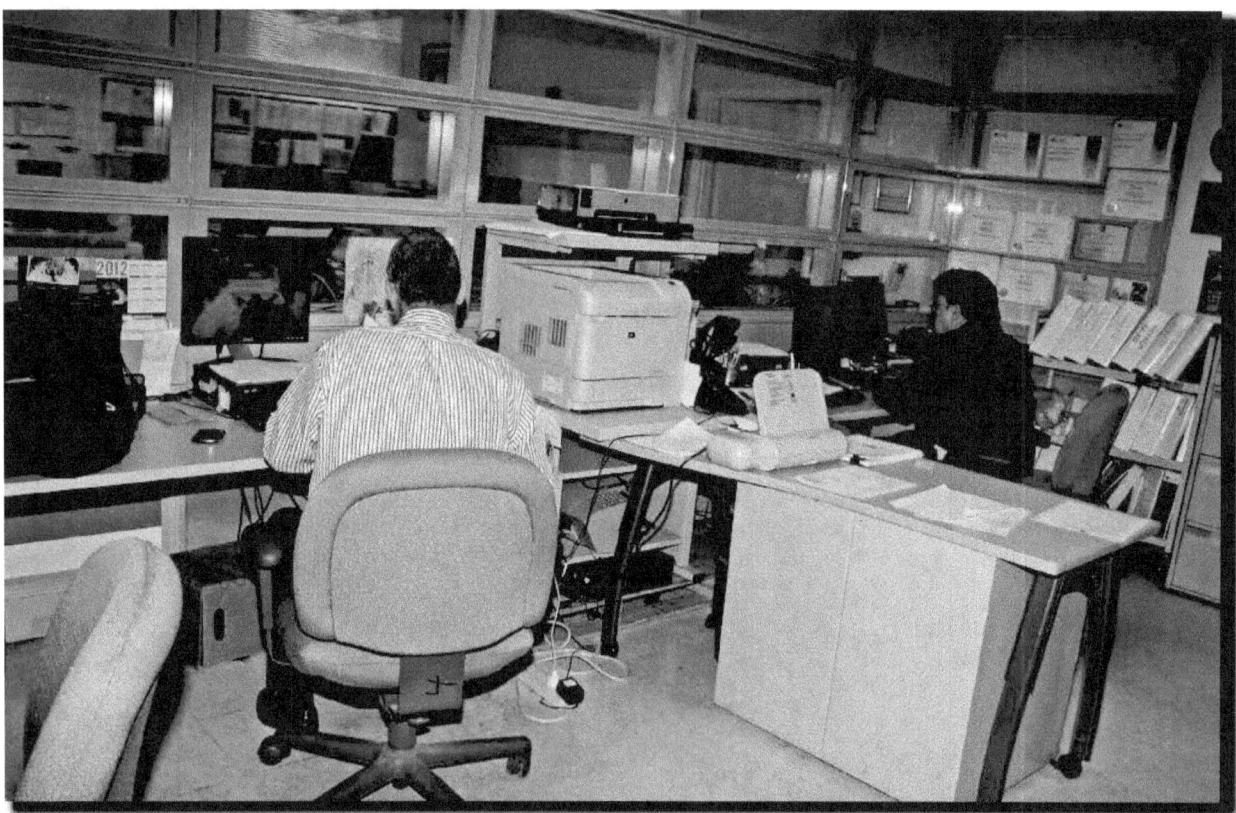

His clients include the largest pharmaceutical companies as well as local smaller members in the arena. Dr. Romeu is currently on board around the clock to make sure that Reliable Research Lab maintains the high expectations this industry demands. Feel free to reach out directly for a personal response to any question at Hugo.Romeu@rerelab.com

Reliable Research Laboratory has become the Industry leader in rapid and secure testing for Clinical Trials. This did not happen overnight, it has taken over 20 years to form the Dream Team of Reliable Of Laboratory Medicine. Our Lab is unique because of the Physicians, Scientists, Technologists and Engineers that make up our in house crew. State of the Art robotic analyzers allow us to perform thousands of tests everyday with the same speed and accuracy as just a few. The menu and staff at Reliable Research Laboratory is extensive and flexible. We can bring in house whatever the study requires. The goal is always the same, to get the tests performed within hours of their arrival into the facility.

Results are reported by fax, secured e-mail, online or in a hard copy.

Research is our forte, and Clinical Laboratory experience is the vehicle which has made us into the very best at what we do.

RRL takes pride in a personal touch. Every Principal Investigator, Study Monitor or Coordinator is encouraged to call us with any question at all.

You can count on us to be a caring partner in achieving your goals.

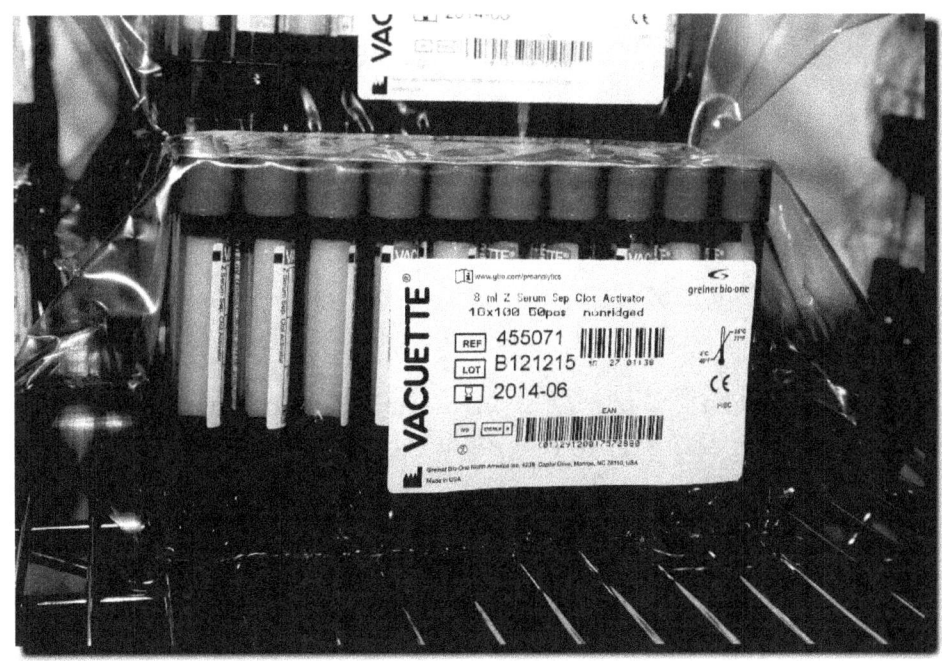

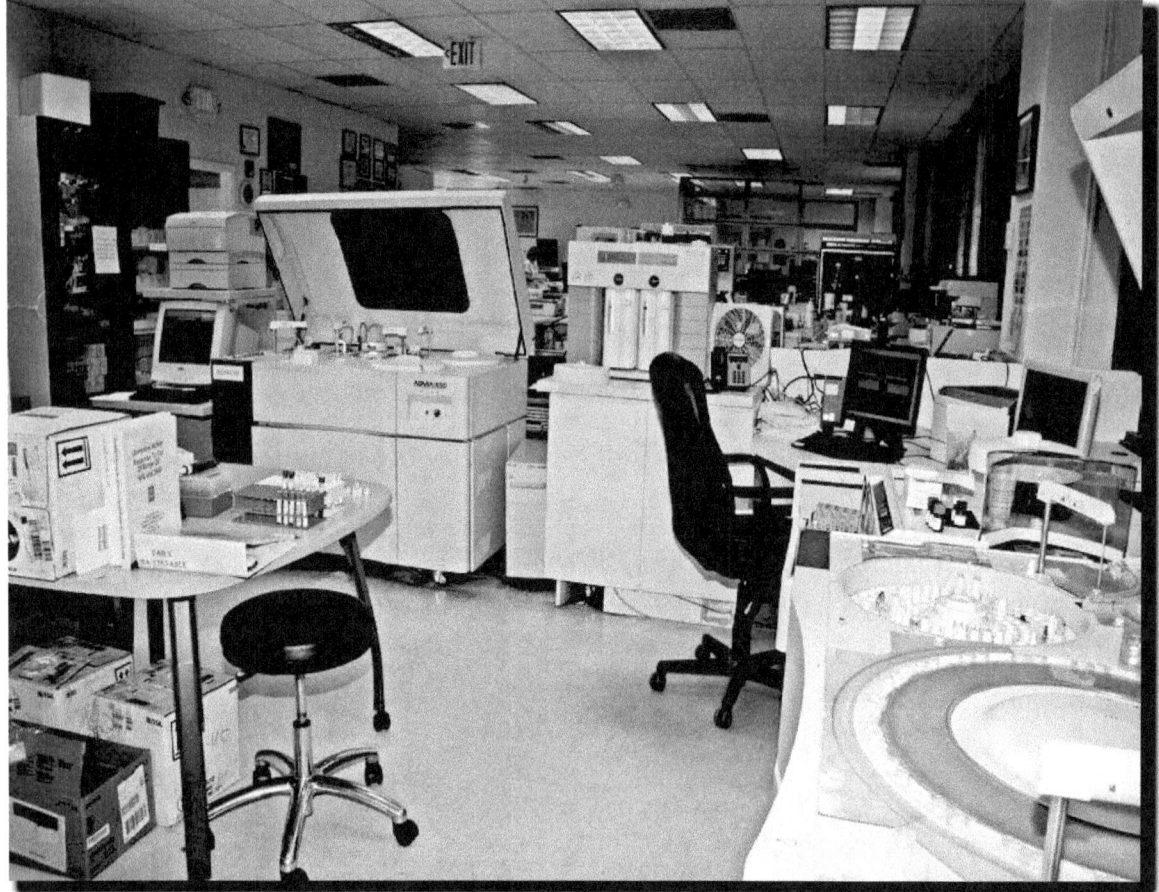

Web portal s are secure and facilitated for immediate and confidential report formats. Only you can see your data, and as soon as it is finished it is visible.

Reliable Research Laboratory is a pharmaceutical research Clinical Laboratory with the infrastructure and personnel to complete the arduous task of reliable and reproducible scientific research. The core participants in our leadership team have been working together for over 24 years.

Together we have completed over 700 studies for all the major global pharmaceutical companies. Our staff of clinicians, pathologists, technologists, is complimented with an in house legal team to oversee the regulatory affairs and any compliance issue.

The Principal owner of Reliable Research Lab is a Pathologist with 32 years of research experience, with direct involvement in every phase of compound development. From pre-clinical trials, protocol and laboratory design to front line investigator work. The entire team was handpicked for their life time of contributions *to the research industry. Every single member of our staff has been involved in hundreds of complex studies of all phases.*

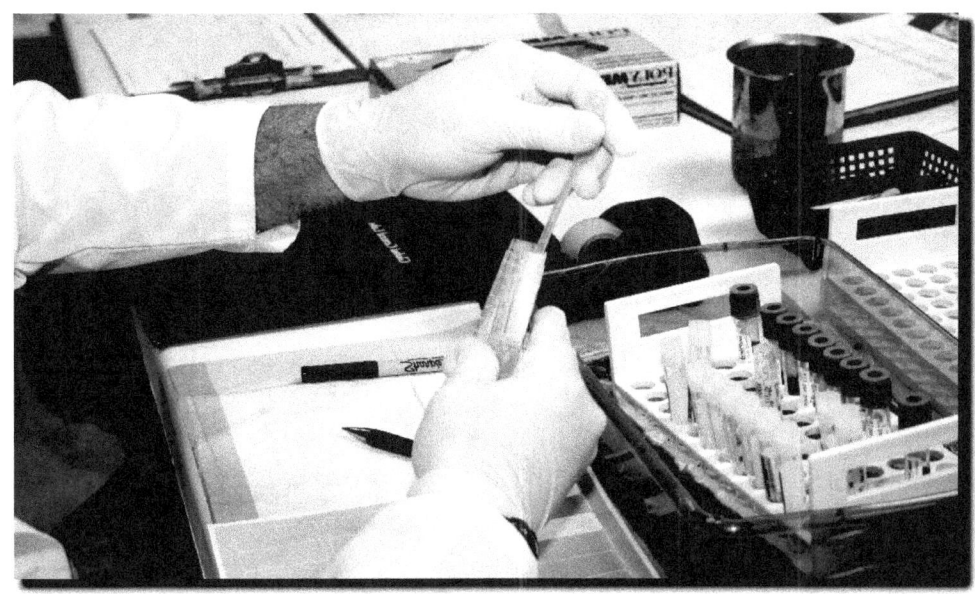

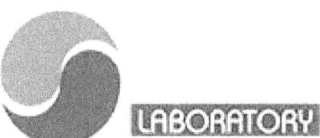

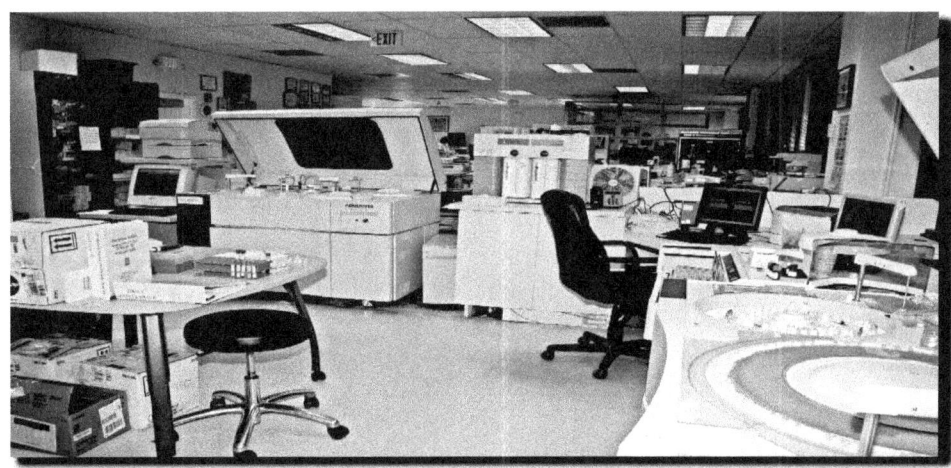

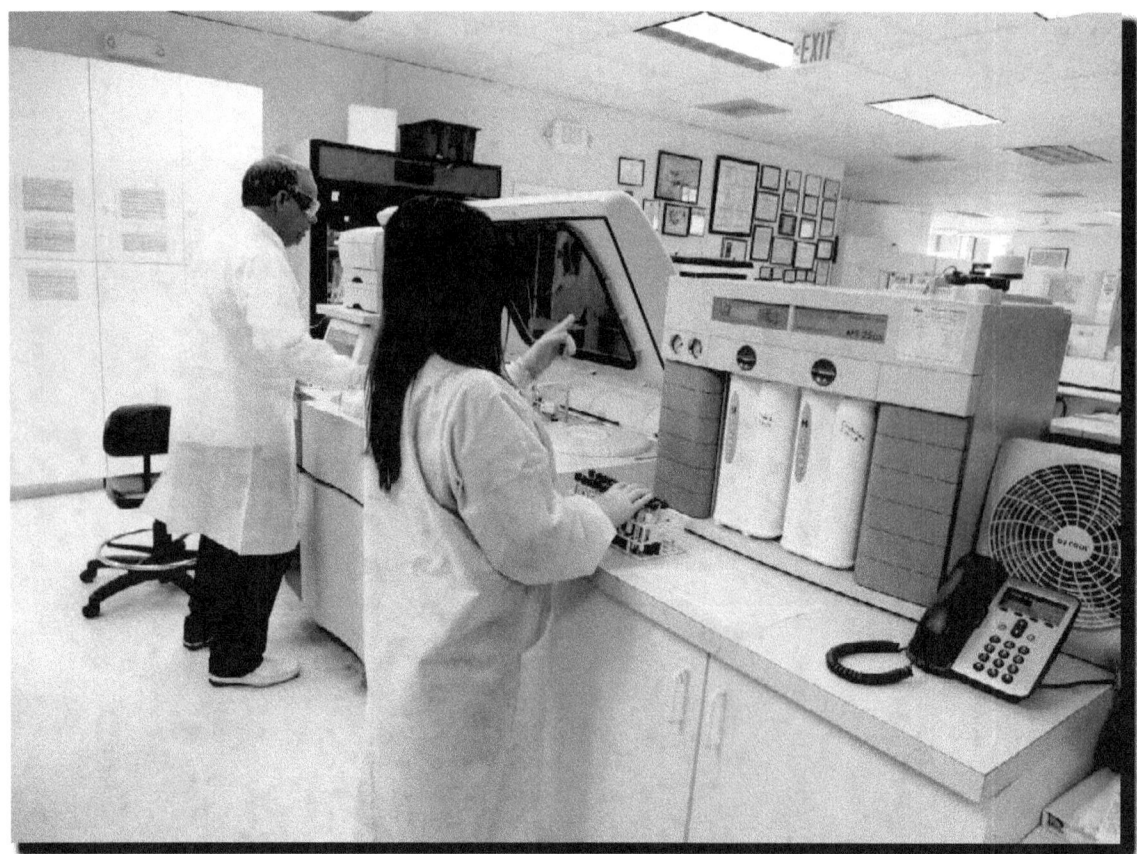

We take pride in our practical and proven experience in the development and establishment of safe medicines which have revolutionized the treatment of the most common afflictions.

Reliable Research Lab is a viable option for any pharmaceutical company because of the infrastructure, extensive training and practical experience of the entire staff.

There are key individuals in leadership roles to oversee the entire operation.

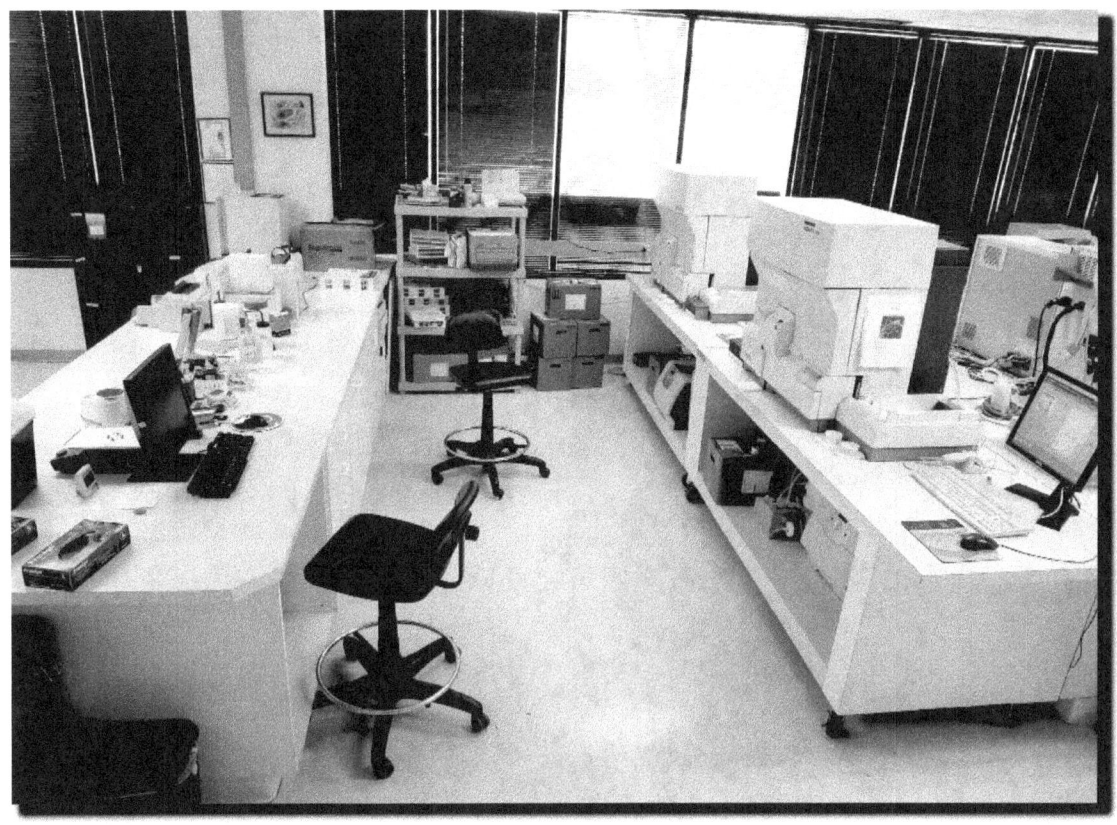

Reliable Research Laboratory is on the forefront of medical research, working with pharmaceutical companies, laboratories and investigators. We have worked on projects to develop new medications, therapeutic and diagnostic modalities, all with a single objective; to cooperate in the advancement of health care.

One of the cornerstones of Reliable Research Laboratory is the expertise in laboratory medicine. We have been involved in the establishment, technical and professional staffing and regulatory guidance for 27 licensed clinical laboratories.

Reliable Research Laboratory also known as ReReLab, provides full service in clinical and anatomic pathology. Our staff is ready to partner with the largest or smallest CRO and or Pharmaceutical Company; to secure an expeditious and reproducible lab data.

One of our strongest facets is the ability to take on a compound in the earliest stages of development; than follow through the late phases. ReReL can assist in the protocol development, especially the areas of laboratory inclusion and exclusion criteria.

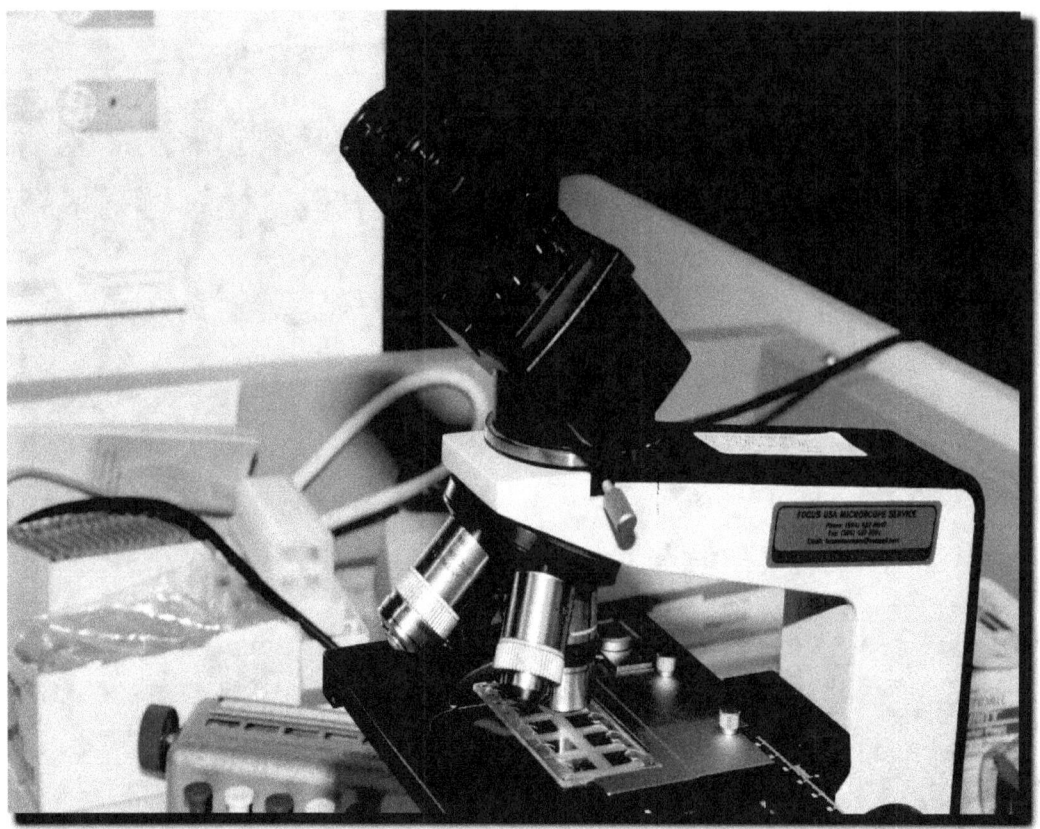

What we do is full-service early phase clinical research: single ascending dose, multiple ascending dose, drug interaction, proof-of-concept, bioequivalence, special populations and therapeutic sub specialties. We test large and small molecules, novel and generic compounds. Our forte is clinical correlation based on review of laboratory data. ReRELab is more than just a site to perform laboratory testing. We are your partners in these studies to secure a safe and successful development of a new or equivalent compound.

What we offer is the data that our clients and sponsors need to make critical decisions when needed: fast, accurate data generated by selecting the most appropriate assay and bio analytical technology. Our experts are ready with the feedback to allow the entire Clinical Team to make the right decisions on how to move forward with their project..

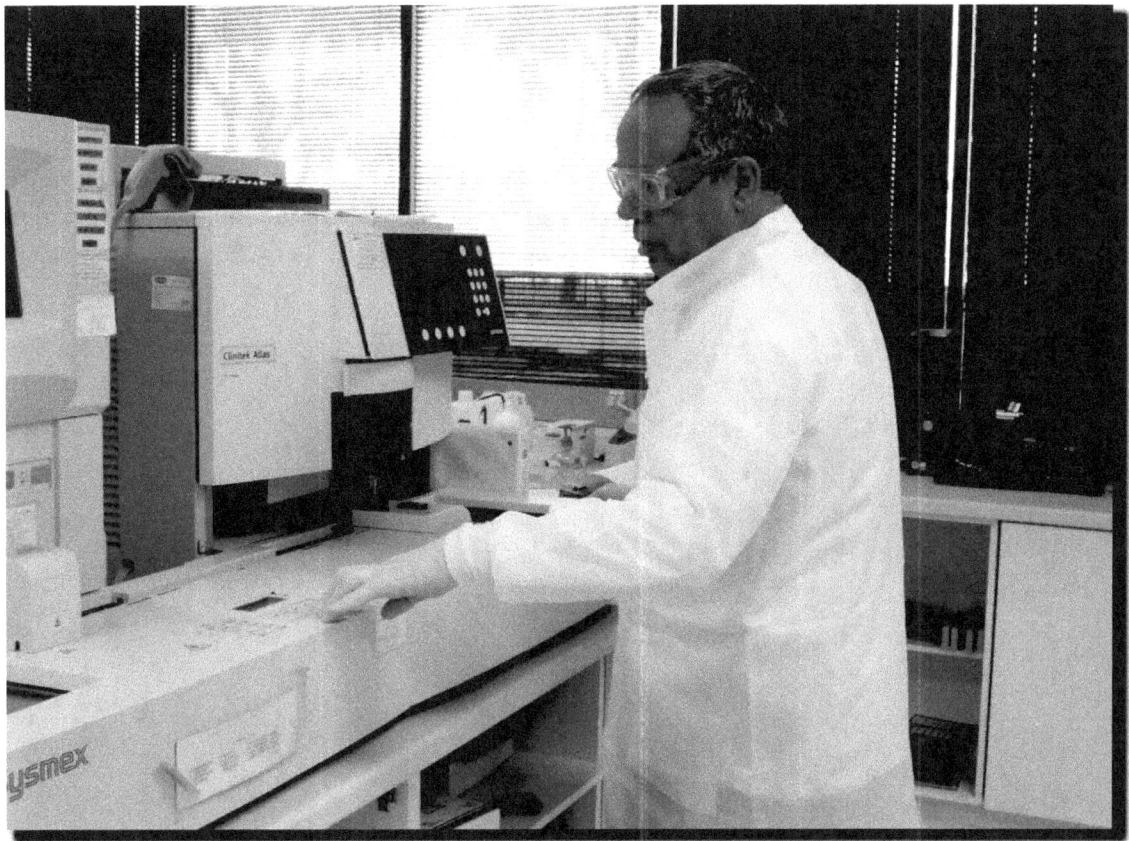

Fast, accurate data generated by selecting the most appropriate assay and bio analytical technology.

We offer a rewarding experience. We're easy to work with and flexible in meeting your needs. If your study has a test which we are not performing, we can bring it in house. Simply because we run open system analyzers which can be programmed to perform the most esoteric requests.
You'll see that for yourself when you meet us. Find out today.

- *Full Service Clinical Laboratory*

- *Security alarmed -70C and -20°C freezers*

- *Spacious procedure areas*

- *State of the Art Equipment*

Why Reliable Research Laboratory ?

We Understand What You Need
And We're the Leaders in Doing It the Way You Want It Done.

Reliable Research Laboratory focuses on full-service early Laboratory Medicine.

Equally important, we focus on each client's specific needs and goals for each specific study. We understand that large pharmaceutical companies, small to mid-size biopharmaceutical firms and generic drug developers all have different needs. And so does each study, although the ultimate goal for all is to develop, as quickly as possible, the data needed to make critical go/no-go decisions with confidence. We'll be happy to talk with you about how our experience and capabilities can help you meet your next early phase challenge. Please contact us at any time.

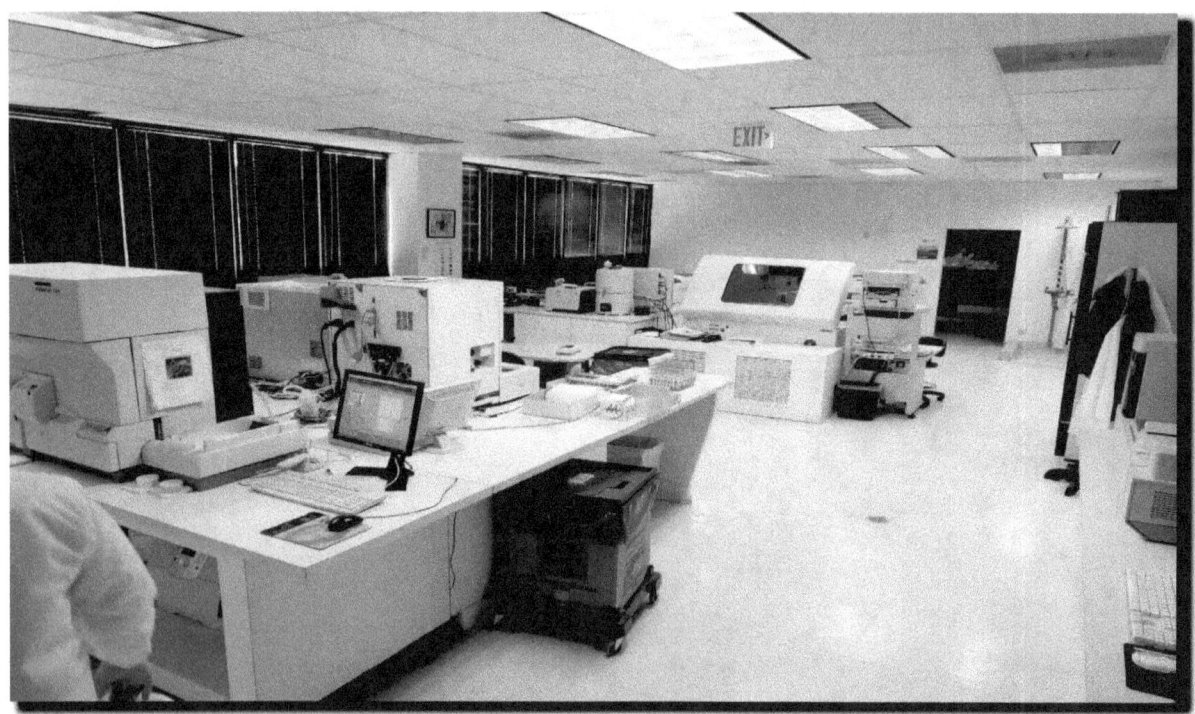

We invite you to discover the ways in which our innovative approaches can cut completion time in half for key types of studies, as well as learn about our customized approaches to serving large pharma, small to mid-size biopharma and generic drug companies – approaches that have made us the industry's leading early phase ReReLab.

Is on the forefront of medical research, working with pharmaceutical companies, laboratories and investigators. We have worked on projects to develop new medications, therapeutic and diagnostic modalities, all with a single objective; to cooperate in the advancement of health care.

One of the cornerstones of Reliable Research Laboratory is the expertise in laboratory medicine. We have been involved in the establishment, technical and professional staffing and regulatory guidance for 27 licensed clinical laboratories. Reliable Research Laboratory provides full service anatomic and clinical pathology consulting.

Reliable Research Laboratory is currently a lead consultant for several of the largest Pharmaceutical Companies.

SERVICES: PRICES ON REQUEST

RELIABLE RESEARCH LABORATORY
(Test Inventory) *

	Test	Specimen
A	Acid Phosphatase Prostatic	R
	Acid Phosphatase Total	R
	Alk. Phosphatase Isoenzymc	R
	Alk. Phos.	R
	Alk.Phosphatase Fractiona rv	R
	Amylase (Serum)	R
	Amylase (24 HR)	U 24HR
	Ammonia = HN3	L
	ANA Titer	R /PPT
	ASO Titer	R
	Acid Fast Smear	Sputum
	Acid Fast Culture S Slain	Sputum
	Acetone (Serum)	R
	Acetaminophen (SND)	R
	Acetylchol Esterase (SND)	R
	Acetylchol Receptor	R
	ACTH	L
	Adeno Virus Titer (SND)	R
	AFB Culture	Sputum
	A Smear Only	
	AldolasE	R
	Aldosterone (Serum)	R
	Aldosterorm (Urine)	u
	Amiodarone	R
	Ant Tromhin	B
	Autogrnous Vaccune	
	Australian Antigen (11,SAg)	R
	Anti DNA	R
	Antigen for Giardia	Stool
	Anlithyroid Peroxid AB	R
	Alpha 1 Antitryptin	R
	ANA = Antinuclear Antibody	R
	Antidiuretic Hormone(ADI)	L
	Antiphospholipid Syndrome (SND)	R
	Antiphosphulipid Antibody (SND)	R
	Asma (Smooth Muscle AB)	R
	Apo E. Genotype	R
	Antimicrosomal Antibody(yhyroid Peroxides Antibody)	R
	ACE (Antiotensin Converting Enzyme) (SND)	R
	AntiSmith (SND)	R
B	B12 by 121	R
	Blood T ype	R-L
	Bilirubin Total	R
	Bilirubin Direct & Indirect	R
	BUN	R
	Biopsy	Biopsy
	Bleeding Time	
	Blood Cultures x 1	Blood Cult.
	BNP (Brain Naturatic Peptide)	PPT (L)
	BMP(Basic Metabolic Panel)	R
	Benze Jones Kapa-- Landa (Urine Electrophoresis)	U 24HR
	Beta 2 Microglobuline	R
	Breath Test =11. Pilory by breath	2 Bags
	Chlantydia Titer (IgM)(IgG)/Chlamydia Culture (SND)	Chlamydia
	Citamegalovirus	R
	Coombs Direct & Indirect	R / L
	Carbon Dioxide	u
	Chloride	R
	Chloride (24HR)	U 24HR
	Chloride Random	u
	Candida	Stool
	CSF Culture	
	Crystalid	
	Cytology Fluid	u
	Cocaine	u

	Test		Specimen
C	Calculus Renal = Stone Analysis		Stone
	Catecholamines		Green
	Catecholamines (24 HR)		U 24HR
	Calculus Analysis		
	Canabinoids		u
	Carbamazepine= Tegretol		R
	CK MB		R
	C- Difficile Antigen		Stool
	C- Difficile Toxin A	(SND)	Stool
	CD4 Absolute	(SND)	L T Yellow
	CD8 Absolute	(SND)	L T Yellow
	CD4 / CD8 Radio		L T Yellow
	Complement C3 / C4		R
	CA 19-9	(SND)	R
	CH50	(SND)	R
	Clele Lucucyte (WBC)		Stool
D	Drug Screen Profile (11)		U
	Drug Screen Profile (7)		U
	DrugScreen Profile (5)		U
	DHEAS	(SND)	R
	DSANA		R
	DHEA		R
	Digoxin By RIA = Lanoxin = Digitalis		R
	Dilantin = Phenitoin		R
	Depakote = Valproid Acid		R
	Drug Screen	(SND)	R
	D. Dimer	(SND)	B
	DHT = Dihidrotestosterone		R
	Dengue	(SND)	R
F	FTA	(SND)	R
	Folic Acid = Folate		R
	Ferritin		R
	Fructosamida	(SND)	R
	Febril Aglutination		R
	Fibrinogen		B
	FSH		R
	Free T3		R
	Free T4		R
	Fungus Culture		Cult.
	Fungus Stain (KOH)	(SND)	Cult.
	Fiftyfibrosis	(SND)	L
	Flu Screen		Cult.
G	Globulin		R
	GFR (Glomeruin Fuction Rate)		R
	G- 6PD (RBC)	(SND)	L
H	HCG Qualitative = Pregnancy Test		R / U
	HCG Quantitative = Pregnancy Test		R
	Homocystine		R
	Herpes Simples Virus Culture	(SND)	Transport.
	Hepatitis C RNA Quant.	(SND)	PPT
	HGB/HCT		L
	HIV 2	(SND)	R
	17 Hydroxyprogesterone		R
	Hepatitis C Ab		R
	17 Hydroxyprogesterone		R
	Hep. C AB		
	Hep. B Viral Load Quant	(SND)	R
	Hep. B Genotype	(SND)	R-PPT
	Hep.B Viral Load	(SND)	R-PPT
	Hep. C RIVA	(SND)	R
	Hep. B Core Igm		R
	Hep. B Total		R
L	LDL		R
	LDH		R
	LDH Isoenzymes		R
	Lipase		R
	Lipoprotein		R
	Lipoprotein Electrophoresic		R
	Lipoprotein Phenotype		R
	LH		R
	LE Floculation		R
	L.E. Prep		R
	L.E. Latex		R
	Liver = Hepatic Function		R
	Lipid Panel=Coronary Risk		R
	Lithium (LI)		R

	Test		Tube
	Lead (Pb)		L
	Lyme Disease	(SND)	R
	Lupus Anticoagulant	(SND)	B
	Leukemia	(SND)	Green-Yellow
	Lupus Analyzer	(SND)	R
	Lupus LE (Lupus Eritromatozo)		R
	Nasal Smear = Eos C		Cult.
	NK Cell	(SND)	3 Yellow
N	Norpramide		R
	Nicotine	(SND)	R
	NMR = VAP	(SND)	NMR Tube
	Phenobarbital		R
	Potassium (K)		R
	Potassium (24 HR)		U 24HR
	Platelet Count		L
	Pregnancy Test (Serum) = HCG		R
	Pregnancy Test (Urine)		u
	PT - Prothombin Time		B
	PTT		B
	PSA = Prostatic Specific Antigen		R
	PSA Free		R
	Phosphorus (P)		R
	Phosphorus Random		u
P	Phosphorus (24 H)		U 24HR
	Protein (Serum)		R
	Protein (24 HR)		U 24HR
	Protein Random		u
	Protein Electrophoresis = Gammopathies		R
	Porphyrins	(SND)	Stool
	Plasmodium		L
	Procainamide		R
	PRGE		R
	Prolactin		R
	Progesterona		R
	Pronestyl		R
	PTH = Parathyroid Hormone		R
Q	Quinidine		R
	Quanriferon — TB Gold		R-L-GY
	Smac 7 = Basic Metabolic Panel		R
	Smac 12 = Comprehensive Metabolic Panel		R
	Smac 18		R
	Smac 22		R
	Smac 26		R
	Sed Rate = ESR		L
	Serum Protein Electrophoesisi		R
	SGOT = AST		R
	SGPT = ALT		R
	Sodium (Na)		R
	Stool Culture		Stool
S	Sickle Cell		L
	Stool for Phophyris	(SND)	Stool
	Synovial Fluid Count		
	SSA		R
	SSB		R
	SCL-70		R
	Strep B Screen (Group A)		Cult
	Stone Analysis		Stone
	Salmonella Titer		R
	Sperm Coun		Semen
	Sperm Culture	(SND)	Semen
	Serotonin	(SND)	R
s	Sinemet		R
	Sex Hormone Vandy Gloobulin		R
	Thyroid Profile (T3-T4-T7)		R
	T3 Uptake		R
	T3 Total		R
	T4		R
	TSH		R
	Triglyceride		R
	Tegretol = Carbamazepin		R
	Throat Culture		Cult.
	Total PSA		R
	Testosterone Free		R
	Testosterone Total		R
T	Thyroglobulin		R

	Transferrine		R
	Trponin		R
	Thin Prep		Thin Prep
	Transferrine		R
	T. Cell	(SND)	Yellow - L
	Theophylline		R
	Toxoplasmosis IgG / IgM		R
	Tyroid Antibody		R
	Thiamine = Vitamin B1	(SND)	R
	Thyroglobulin Antibody		R
	Thyroperoxide		R
	Trasglutaminace		R
V	Vaginal Culture		Cult.
	Varicela Titer IgC		R
	Vancomycin Through		R
	Vancomycin Peak		R
	Valproic Acid Total = Depakote		R
	Vitamin BI = Thiamine	(SND)	R (frozen)
	Valproic Free	(SND)	R
	Vanillymandolia AC		U 24HR
	Vitamin D		R
	Varicela IgM	(SND)	R
	Viral Culture	(SND)	
	Viral Load	(SND)	PL / L
	Vit. D 25 I Hydroxy		R
	Vit. B1	(SND)	R
	Vit. B6	(SND)	L
	Vit. K	(SND)	Green
	Vit. D 125 Dihydroxy	(SND)	R
	Vit A (Retinol)	(SND)	R
Z	Zolof		R
	Zinc	(SND)	Navy Blue

* Price on request

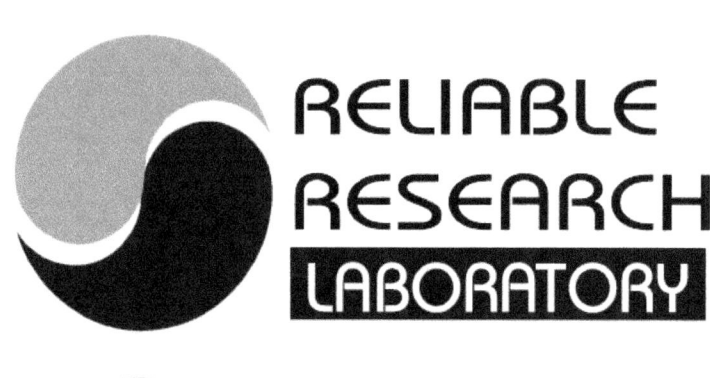

PharmRCE USA
     Dr. Hugo Romeu M.D.

PHARM RCE USA

dr.hugoromeu@yahoo.com

PharmRCE

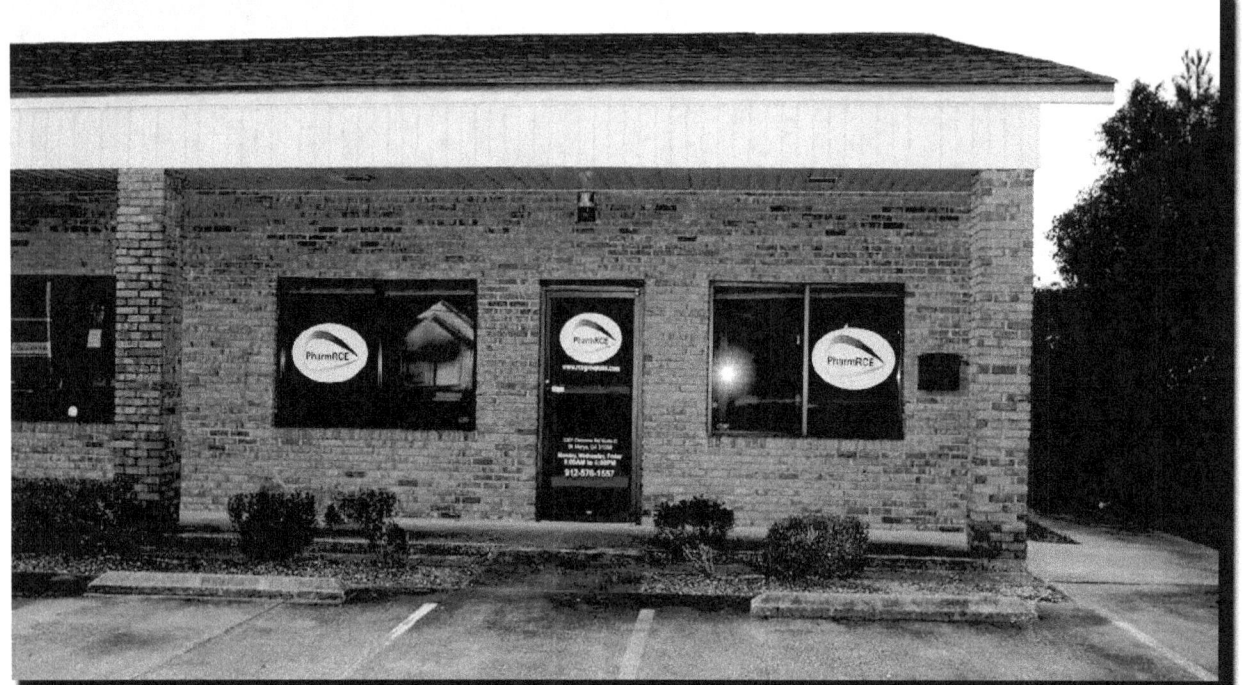

PharmRCE USA

2201 Osborne Road, Saint Marys, Camdem County Georgia 31558

1-(912) 510 4900

PharmRCE USA

PharmRCE USA, is a Wholesale pharmaceutical distributor. We are a service oriented company, which pays close attention to the needs of the individual and the larger company. Our focus is providing a service to USA and Latin America.

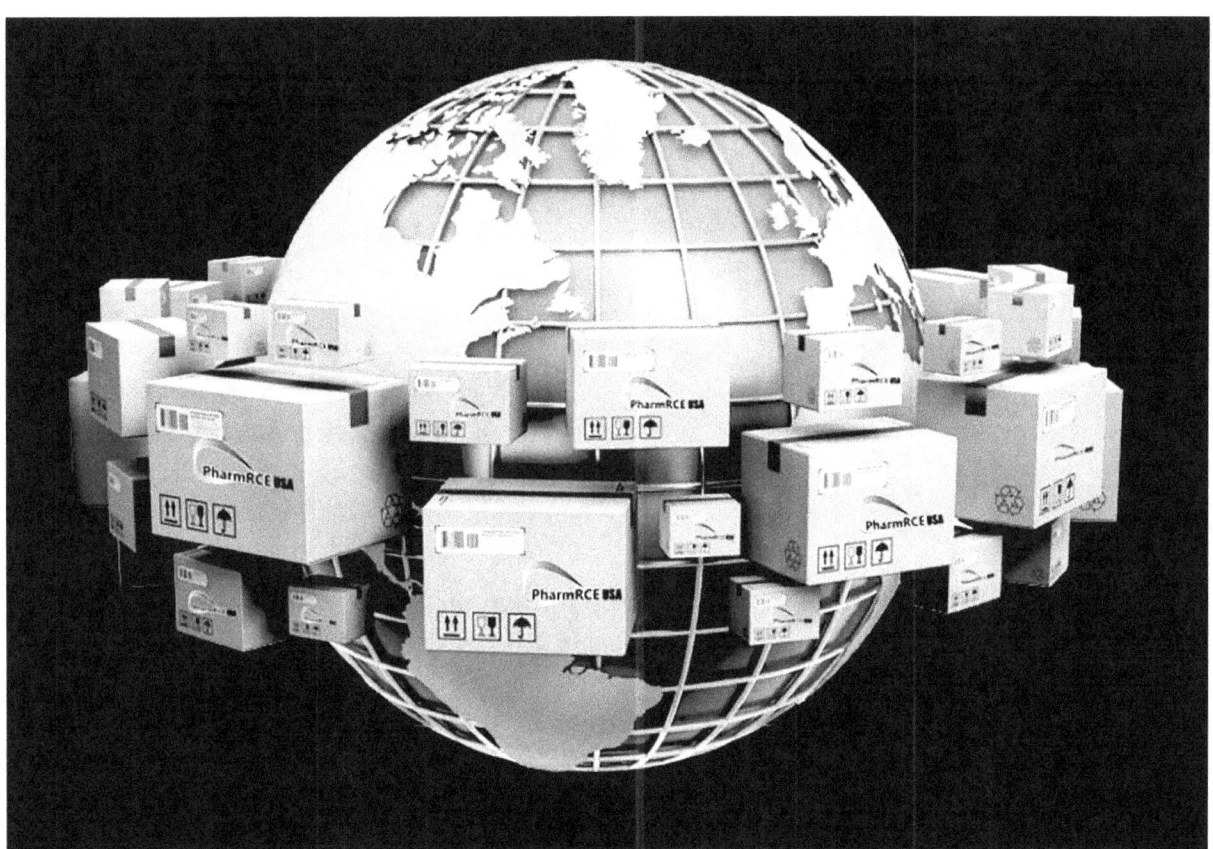

Pharm RCE USA, llc is located in the quaint town of St. Mary's Georgia, close to the Florida and Georgia northeast state border.

This is a wholesale pharmaceutical company specialized in difficult to acquire over the counter products, cosmetics, beauty creams, fillers and entire lines for the anti-aging industry.

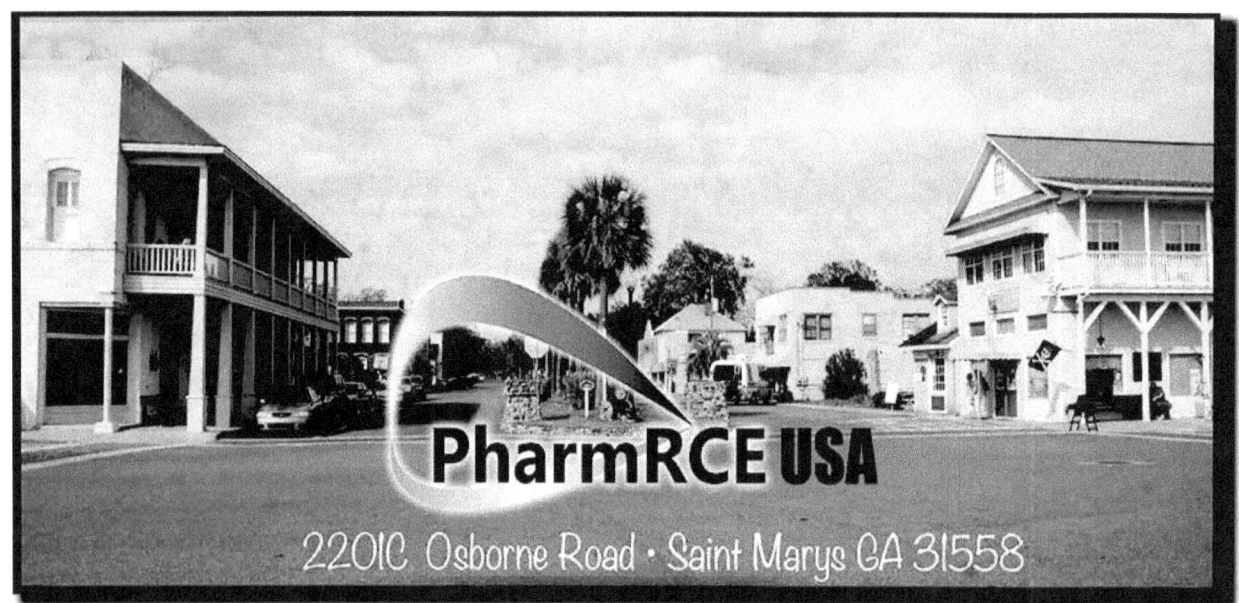

Our mother and sister companies service the pharmaceutical industry at all levels; from phase 1 ,2,3,4 clinical research, pharmacokinetics, clinical laboratory testing, as well as protocol development.

All studies have some commonalities, like comparing a new compound to existing and approved products.

At Pharm RCE USA, we cater to the Clinical Research Organizations performing studies which need to purchase bioequivalent pharmaceuticals for their ongoing and upcoming studies.

Furthermore we aggressively pursue the purchase of short dated medications, and generics, therefore offering our clients significant discounts.

An added benefit of doing business with us is the availability of products for the Latin American market through Pharm RCE in Mexico.
For further information please contact us at

info@pharmrceusa.com

PharmRCE USA Located in Saint Marys,GA and is a company dedicated to the distribution of products related to the health area and our main objective is not only to get leads, but keep them satisfied, only offering a service compared to the quality of the products we offer.

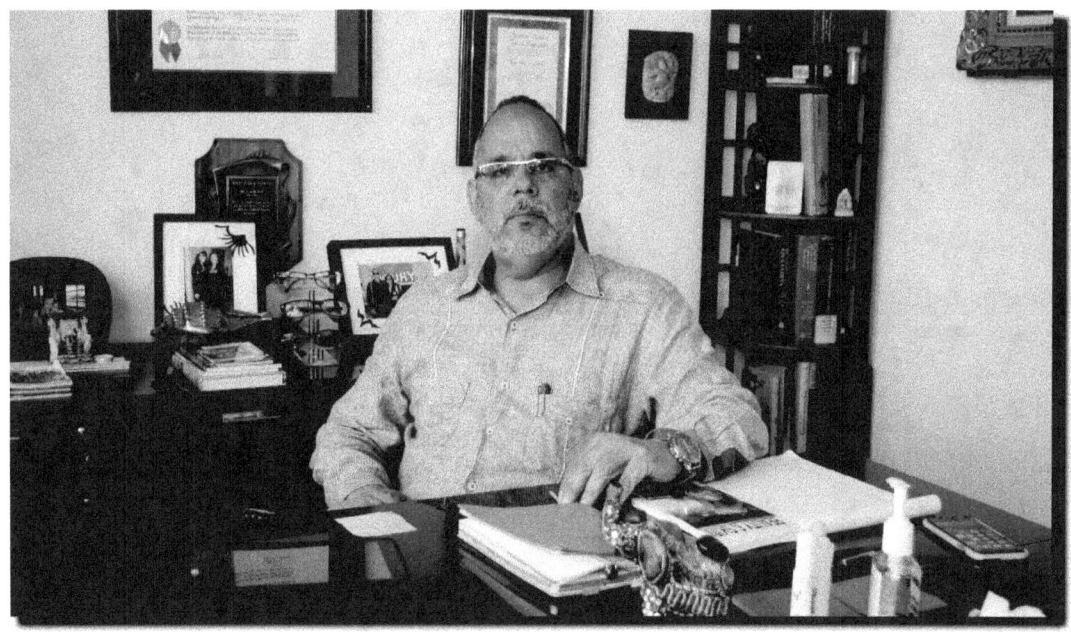

The wholesale provides a number of advantages, a wholesale-client that allows advantageous transactions within a framework of respect and cooperation, achieving better deals, better prices and better terms of delivery relationship is established, taking into account the greater the quantity, the price will be decreased.

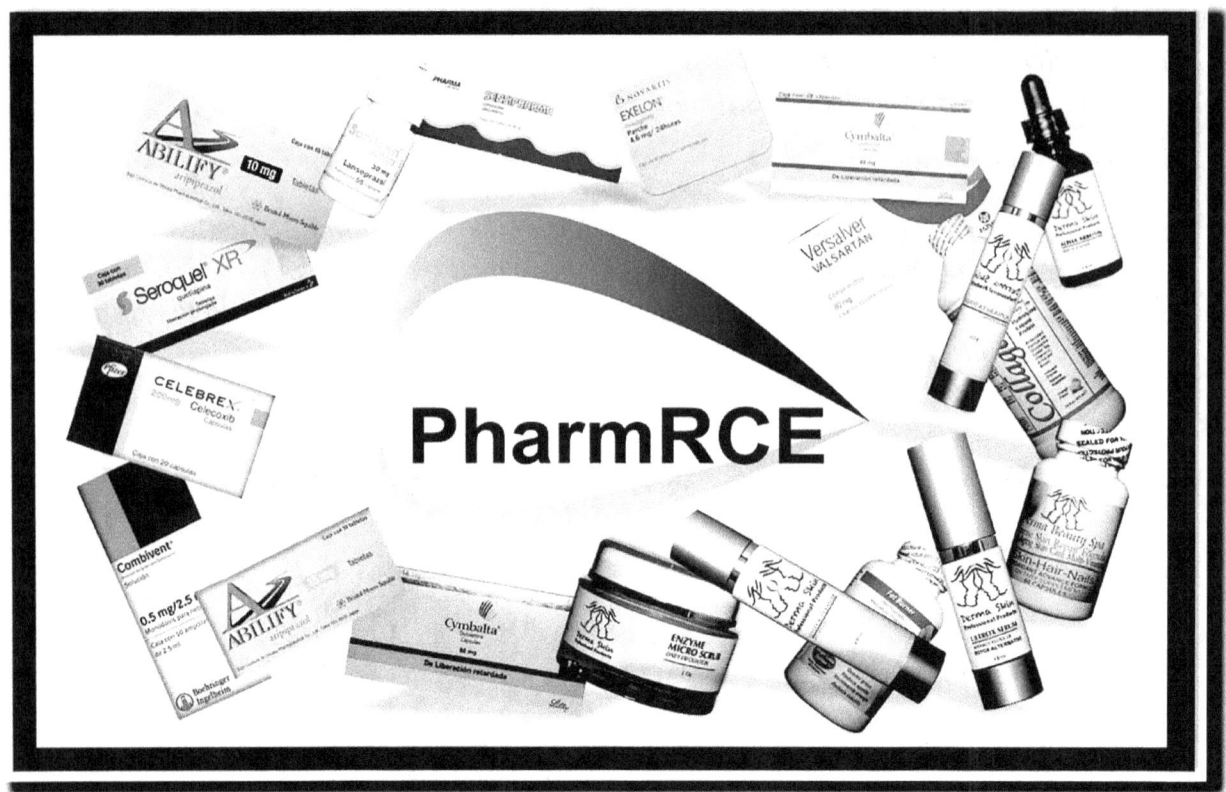

It bought in quantities, managed to decrease not only the price of the product but the cost of handling and shipping, thus achieving an attractive investment, with the margin sufficient to enable substantial gains, even offering consumers a lower price than you're used , something that will give your business a competitive market support that will guarantee the current sales without doubt be reflected in increased customer base.

PharmRCE USA is at disposal, without obligation, to offer you the price of the products you need in the quantities required, we are in the position to negotiate directly with you to reach a point of compromise that satisfies both.

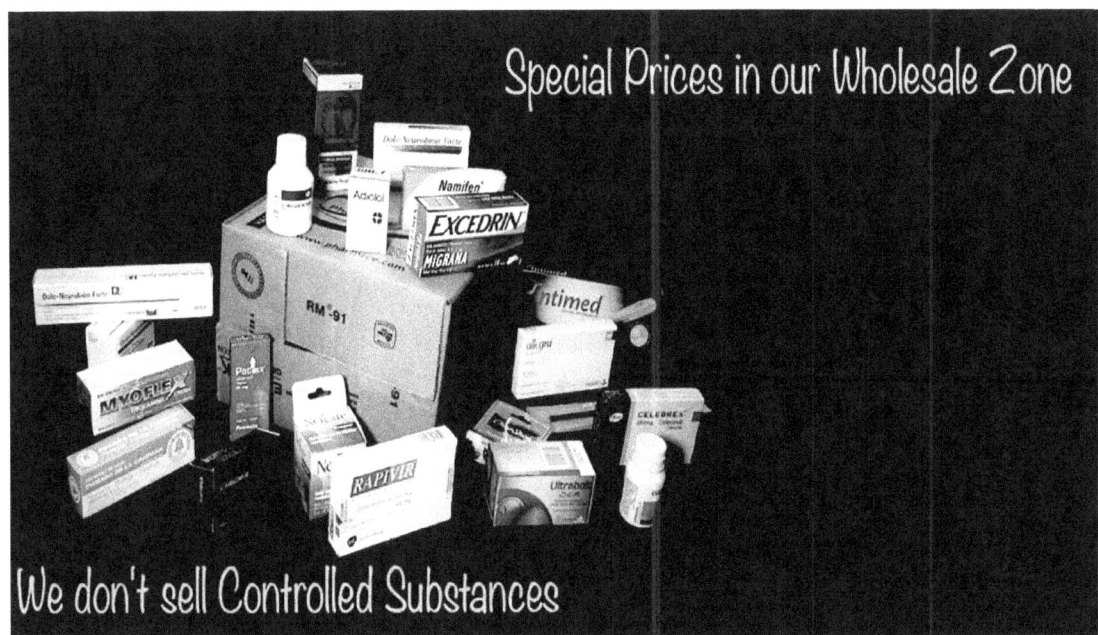

The right time is now here we are waiting for you to contact us.

info@pharmrceusa.com

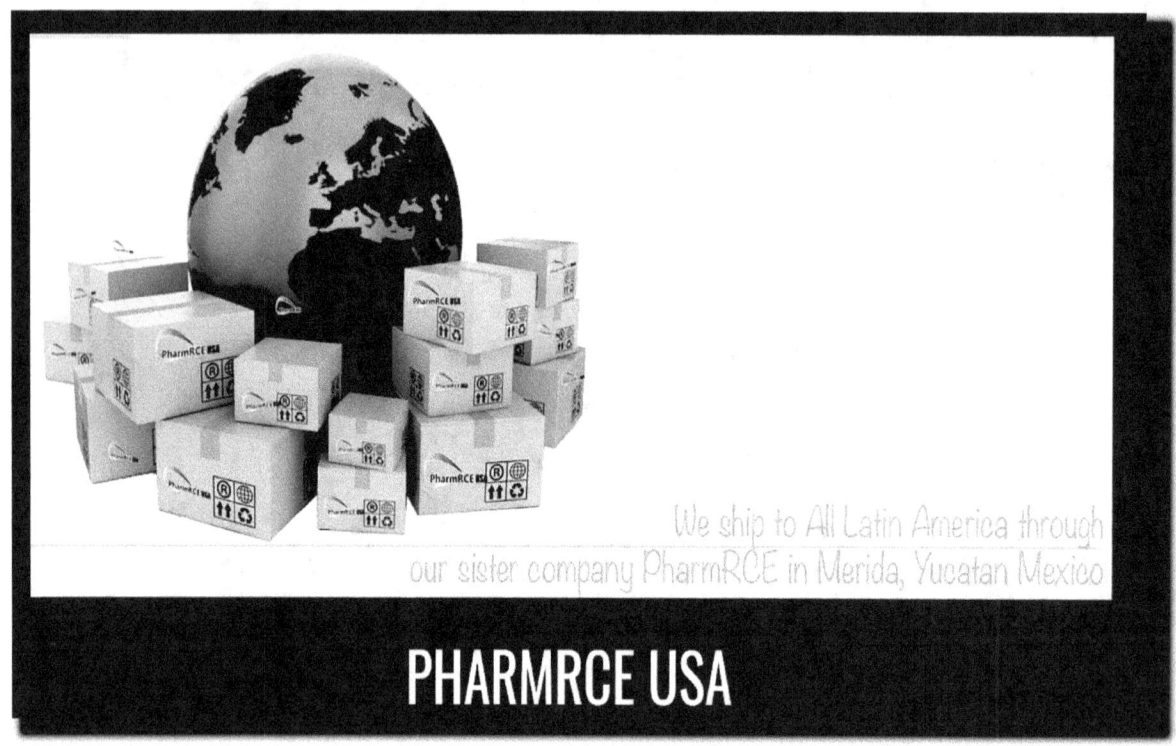

Ask for the alphabetical list of the products we have available to bid wholesale. You can find in our website
www.pharmrceusa.com

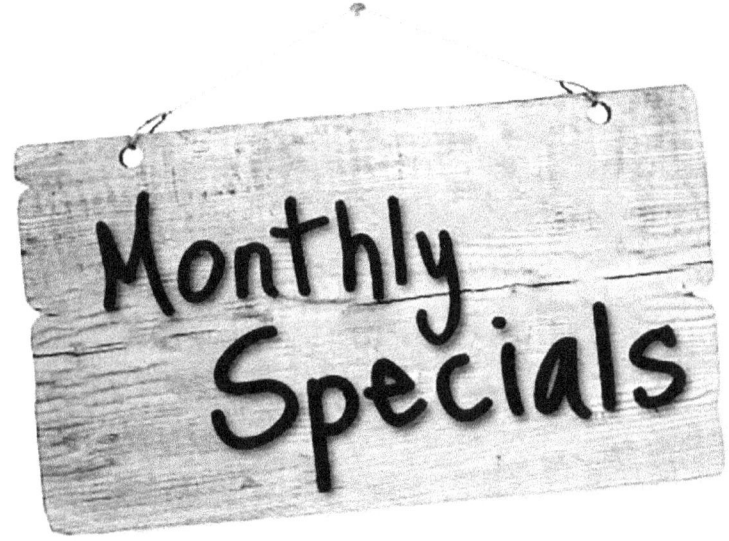

Always we have special sales, I will show as a sample
December 2016 ...

PharmRCE USA

2201-C Osborne Road
Saint Marys, GA 3155 • ☎ (912) 576-1557

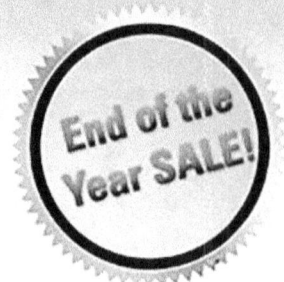

End of the Year SALE!

TYLENOL 25 X-STRENGHT	50 Pouches 2 Caplets	$12.05
ADVIL PM 2S	50 Pouches 2 Caplets	$15.39
ALEVE CAPLET 1S	48 Pouches 1 Caplet	$12.65
CLARITIN ALERGY TABLETS SINGLES	1 Pq 25 Each	$20.35
PEPTO BISMOL 4Oz	1 Dozen	$28.60
NYQUIL COLD & FLUE 8Oz	1 Dozen	$73.65
DAYQUIL COLD & FLUE 8Oz	1 Dozen	$73.65

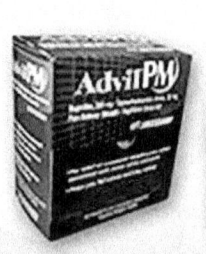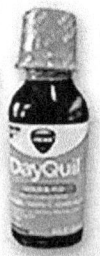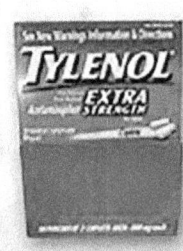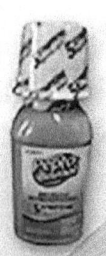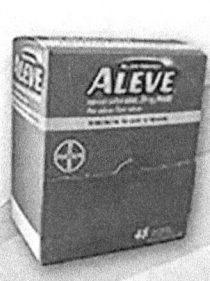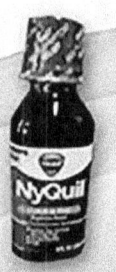

TROJAN BLACK MAGNUM	48 BOXES 3 EACH	$67.38
TROJAN GREY ULTRA THIN	48 BOXES 3 EACH	$67.38
TROJAN RED ENZ NON-LUBRICATED	48 BOXES 3 EACH	$49.95
TROJAN DARK BLUE ARMOR SPERMICIDAL	48 BOXES 3 EACH	$67.38
TROJAN BROWN ULTRA RIBBED	48 BOXES 3 EACH	$67.38
TROJAN PURPLE HER PLEASURE SENSATION	48 BOXES 3 EACH	$67.38
TROJAN FIRE ICE FIRE ICE	48 BOXES 3 EACH	$81.90
TROJAN MAGNUM THIN	48 BOXES 3 EACH	$81.90
TROJAN BLUE ENZ LUBRICATED	48 BOXES 3 EACH	$62.72

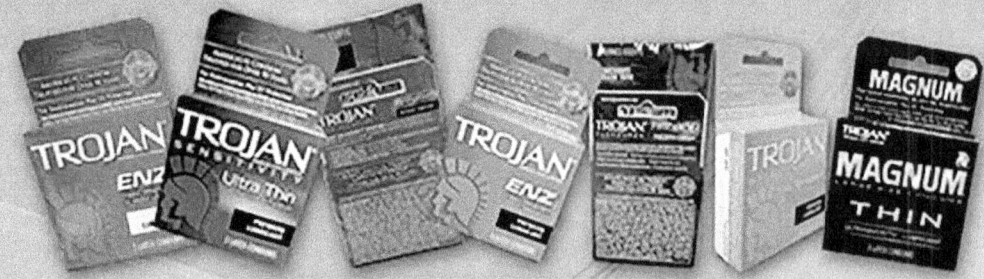

www.pharmrceusa.com

info@pharmrceusa.com   orders@pharmrceusa.com

PharmRCE USA
2201-C Osborne Road
Saint Marys, Ga 31558
(912) 576 1557

PharmRCE USA

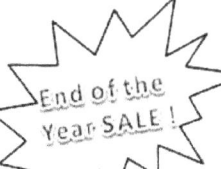

End of the Year SALE !

TYLENOL 2S X-STRENGHT	50	Pouches	2	Caplets	$12.05
ADVIL PM 2S	50	Pouches	2	Caplets	$15.39
ALEVE CAPLETS 1S	48	Pouches	1	Caplets	$12.65
CLARITIN ALLERGY TABLETS SINGLES	1	Pq	25	Each	$20.35
PEPTO BISMOL 4OZ	1	Dozen			$28.60
NYQUIL COLD & FLU 8OZ	1	Dozen			$73.65
DAYQUIL COLD & FLU 8OZ	1	Dozen			$73.65

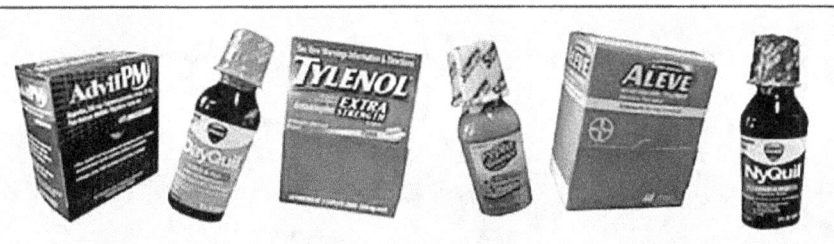

Trojan Black Magnum	48	Boxes	3 each	$67.38
Trojan Grey Ultra Thin	48	Boxes	3 each	$67.38
Trojan Red Enz Non-Lubricated	48	Boxes	3 each	$49.95
Trojan Dark Blue Armor-Spermicidal	48	Boxes	3 each	$67.38
Trojan Brown Ultra Ribbed	48	Boxes	3 each	$67.38
Trojan Purple Her Pleasure-Sensations	48	Boxes	3 each	$67.38
Trojan Fire-Ice Fire-ice	48	Boxes	3 each	$81.90
Trojan Magnum Thin Magnum Thin	48	Boxes	3 each	$81.90
Trojan Blue Enz Lubricated	48	Boxes	3 each	$62.72

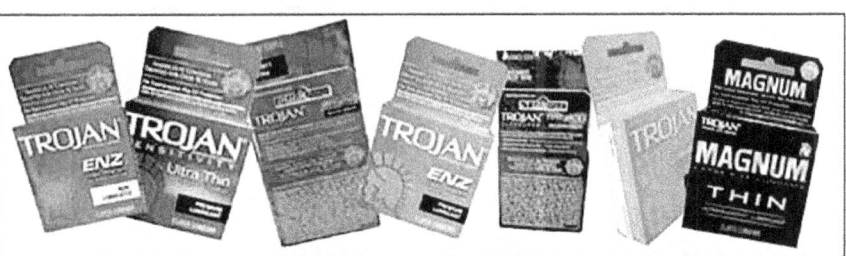

www.farmrceusa.com

info@pharmrceusa.com   orders@pharmrceusa.com

PharmRCE USA, tiene una Empresa hermana, PharmRCE México, radicada en Mérida, Yucatán.

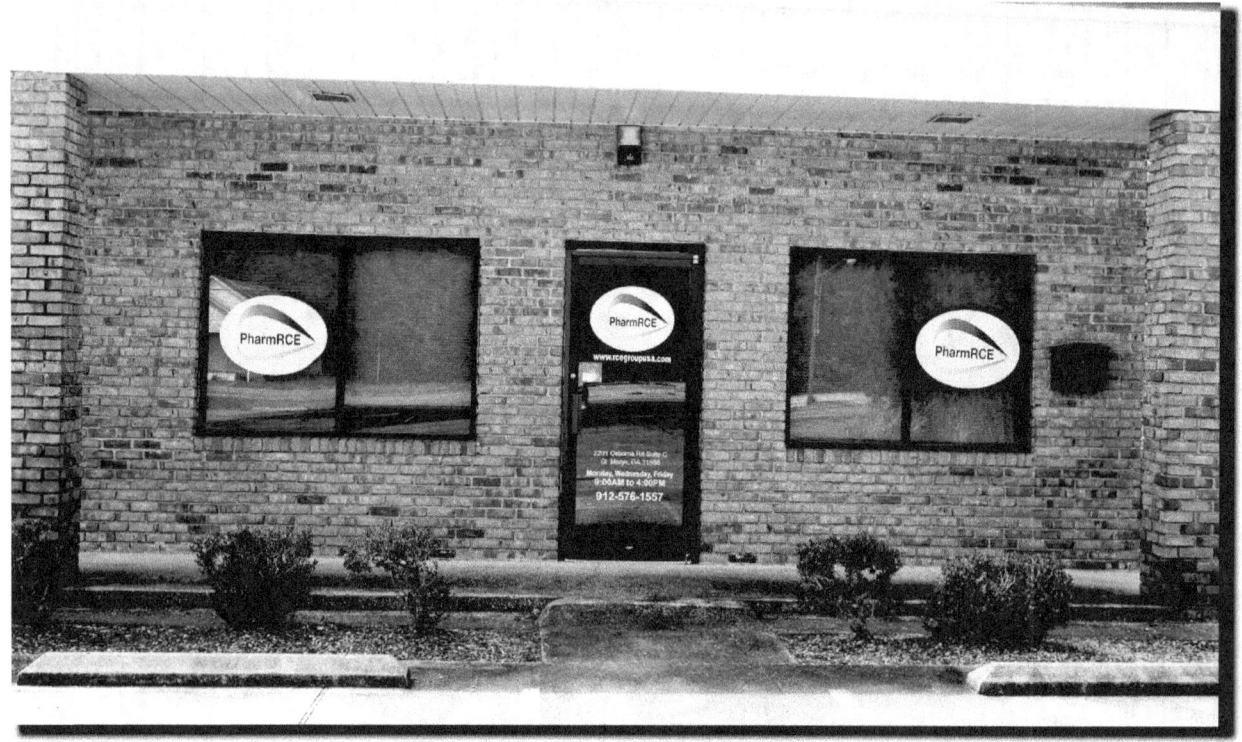

Calle 60 #323A, Colonia Centro, Mérida, Yucatán. México 97000
Phone: Cell 1-(305)-627 3703   (999) 287 3142
www.pharmrce.com.mx

PharmRCE USA, is part of the RCE Group USA

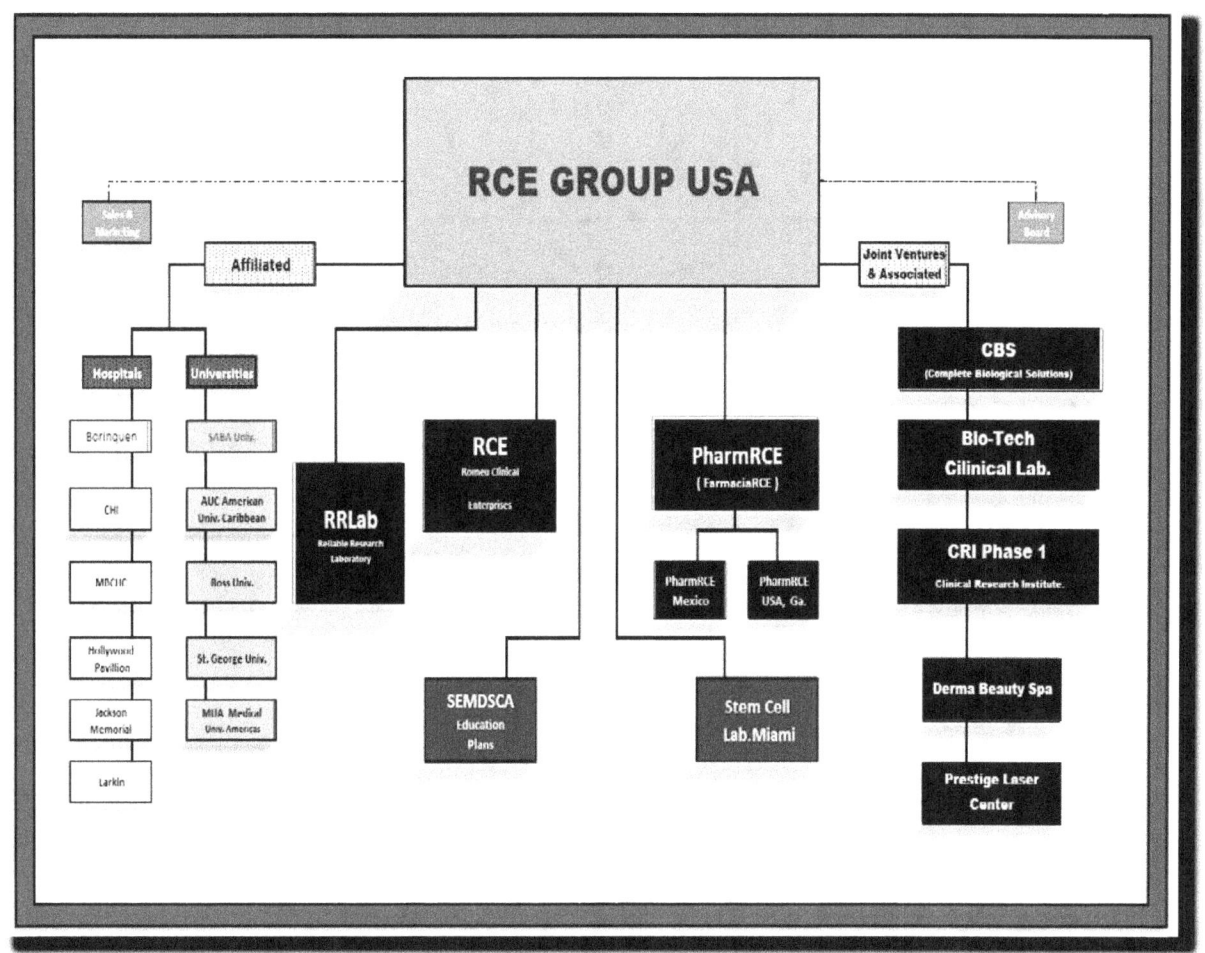

ORGANIGRAMA RCE GROUP USA

PHARMRCE USA

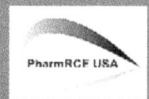

Sample of products over the counter
we are promoting

1		MOTRIN IB 20s Liquid Gel
2		CHILDREN ADVIL 4oz Liquid
3		BAYER ASPIRIN Tablets 24s
4		BENGAY GreaseLess 2oz Tube
5		BENGAY Vanishing 2oz Tube
6		TYLENOL XS 10ct Tablets carded
7		TYLENOL XS 10ct Tablets Counter display

8		TYLENOL PM Caplets caplets 24s
9		TYLENOL Infant Drops 1oz Grape
10		CHILD TYLENOL 4oz Cherry Suspension
11		TYLENOL caplet 24s Extra-strength
12		ADVIL 10ct Tablets
13		ADVIL CAPLETS 24ct
14		ADVIL TABLETS 24ct
15		ADVIL PM Capletes 20ct

16		EXCEDRIN Caplets 24s Extra Strength
17		EXCEDRIN MIGRAINE 24ct caplets
18		EXCEDRIN PM tab 24s Tablets
19		ALEVE tablets 24s
20		ALEVE Caplets 24s
21		MOTRIN CHILDREN 4oz Suspension Berry
22		MOTRIN INFANT DROPS 0.5oz Berry

23		MOTRIN PM Caplets 20ct
24		GENERIC EXCEDRIN REGULAR Tablets 50x2s
25		BENADRYL GENERIC Tablets 50x1s
26		IMODIUM GENERIC Tablets 50x1s

27		TYLENOL SINUS Generc Tablets 50x2s
28		XXXXXXXXXXXXX
29		GENERIC TYLENOL PM Tablets 34x2s
30		ALLERGY/SINUS 50x2pk CompareTo TYLENOL ALLERGY
31		(USA) VICKS VapoRub 1.76oz
32		VICKS COUGH DROPS Cherry box of 20
33		VICKS COUGH DROPS Menthol box of 20
34		Dristan Nasal spray 1/2oz Long Lasting

35		ALKA SELTZER PLUS DAY-TIME 6ct
36		ALKA SELTZER PLUS NIGHT-TIME 6ct
37		AFRIN nasal spray 15ml
38		TYLENOL COLD 24s Multi-Symptoms
39		ROBITUSSIN Children 4oz Cough Syrop
40		THERA FLU 6s (green) Nasal Congestion Cold
41		THERAFLU POWDER 6s LIPTON MultiSymptom (yel)
42		THERAFLU POWDER 6s DayTime Cough Cold

43		DAYQUIL LIQUICAPS 16ct
44		NYQUIL LIQUICAPS 16ct
45		ZZZQUIL SLEEP AID 6oz NightTime
46		NYQUIL 8oz Liquid Cold + Flu
47		NYQUIL COLD + FLU 8oz cherry
48		DAYQUIL 8oz Liquid Cold + Flu
49		TYLENOL Daytime Multi/Symptoms Cold 8oz
50		TYLENOL NightTime Multi/Symptoms Cold 8oz

51		TYLENOL COLD+FLU Caplets 24s
52		PEPTO BISMOL Liquid 4oz Original
53		PEPTO BISMOL Liquid 8oz Original
54		IMODIUM AD caps 6s
55		MILK OF MAGNESIA PHILLIPS reg 4oz
56		ROLAIDS Tablets 10s Fruit Box of 12x10
57		ROLAIDS Tablets 12s Peppermint Box of 12x12

58		ZANTAC 75 4s Acid Reducer tablets
59		EX-LAX PILLS 8ct Regular strength Laxative
60		GAS-X SOFTGEL 10ct Extra Stength AntiGas
61		GAS-X TABLETS 18s Chewable
62		TUMS singles box/12 Xtra-strength Asst fruit
63		TUMS singles box/12 Peppermint
64		TUMS singles box/12 Berry
65		J+J 1st AID KIT 12ct

66		J+J PLASTIC Band-Aid 3/4 X 3in 8s
67		J+J PLASTIC Band-Aid 30ct Assorted Sizes
68		J+J PLASTIC Band-Aid 60ct 3/4x3inch
69		NEOSPORIN ointment 0.5 oz Tube
70		ACE TYPE bandage 2inch elastic
71		ACE type Bandage 3inch elastic
72		Adhesive TAPE 1inch X 5yds carded
73		2ft GUAZE BANDAGE 2 inch white

74		GAUZE BADAGE 3inch Hangable
75		Plastic strips 10ct Generic Bandaid
76		IODINE 1oz Liquid
77		LUCKY FIRST-AID KIT 42 Items (Travel Kit)
78		LUCKY BAND-AID 100s Assorted sizes
79		LUCKY HYDROCORTISONE Cream 0.5oz Tube
80		LUCKY A + D OINTMENT 1.25oz for diaper rash

81		LUCKY PAIN RELIEF Cream 1.5oz Tube
82		LUCKY ANTI-ITCH Relief Ointment 1.25oz
83		LUCKY TOOTHACHE Relief Gel 0.5oz
84		LUCKY BACITRACIN Ointment 0.5oz Anti-Biotc
85		NOXZEMA creme 2oz
86		VASELINE PJ 1.75oz Jars (USA)
87		VASELINE PJ 3.75oz Jars (USA)
88		LUCKY PetroleumJelly 6oz jar

89		LUCKY BODY LOTION 20oz Aloe
90		LUCKY COCOA BUTTER Body Cream 8oz
91		LUCKY COCOA BUTTER BODY LOTION 20oz.
92		LUCKY LOTION 15oz Vitamin E
93		VISINE 0.5oz regular
94		VISINE 0.28oz Carded Advance relief
95		Clear eyes 0.2oz Pocket pal
96		Trojan-ENZ lub 3s (Blue box) 93050
97		REG Trojan 3s (Red box)

98		RIBBED Trojan 3s (Brown box)
99		TROJANs Spermcidl (dark blue box)
100		TROJANs 3s Ultrathin lubricated (grey box)
101		TROJAN ECSTASY 3s Condoms
102		TROJAN Magnum 3s Thin Condoms
103		MAGNUM -CHARGED- 3s TROJAN intensified
104		TROJANs 3s Magnum Lubricated
105		XL TROJANs Magnum 3s
106		MAGNUM SINGLES 40ct Box Display Lubricated

107		MAGNUM SINGLES 48ct Box Display Lubricated
108		TROJANs 3s Her Pleasure
109		TROJANs 3s Pleasure Pack 3s
110		TROJANs 3s Fire + Ice 3s
111		TROJAN BARESKIN 3s Lubricated
112		TROJAN MAGNUM RIBBED 3s
113		TROJAN BARESKING 3s Magnum

StemCell Miami
Dr. Hugo Romeu M.D.

STEM CELL MIAMI

dr.hugoromeu@yahoo.com

Stem Cell

Our Laboratory **Stem Cell Laboratory** is committed to excellence in processing and cryogenically storing your child's cord blood. Using state-of-the-art equipment and highly qualified personnel, we ensure the highest quality standard is upheld thus providing the best possible service for our clients. Our laboratory is based in the dynamic city of Miami, by making South Florida our home we have access to a very diverse clientele providing us with the unique opportunity of working in a world-class city known for being the gateway to international communities.

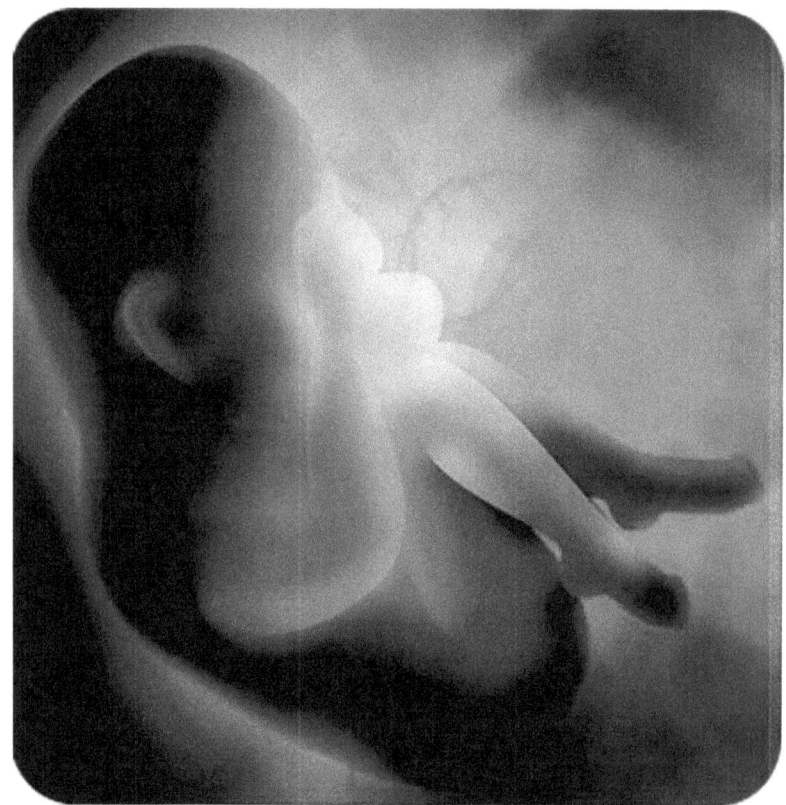

Our highly qualified laboratory director who has overseen tens of thousands of processed cord blood units, and has also released units for transplant supervises our laboratory. The laboratory technicians are highly experienced in processing and storing cord blood.
Our clients can rest assured that their child's processed cord blood will be stored under proper temperatures at all times. Our cryogenic storage devices are generators and back-up nitrogen tanks in the facility.

Our Processing

Your child's cord blood can be shipped to our facility immediately after the collection has taken place. All the necessary materials needed for the processing of your child's cord blood will arrive at our laboratory under controlled conditions in order to guarantee the safeguard of the unit. We process our client's cord blood using a widely accepted and validated volume reduction system. This system is very efficient in recovering a high number of total nucleated cells needed for transplant.

As part of our processing procedures we will test the cord blood samples for cell viability and total Stem Cells using flow cytometer. The cord blood will also be tested to determine the sterility and total nucleated cell count (TNC). The maternal blood collected at the time of delivery will be tested for infectious diseases and blood type. All our processing and testing takes place under Strict Quality Control conditions.

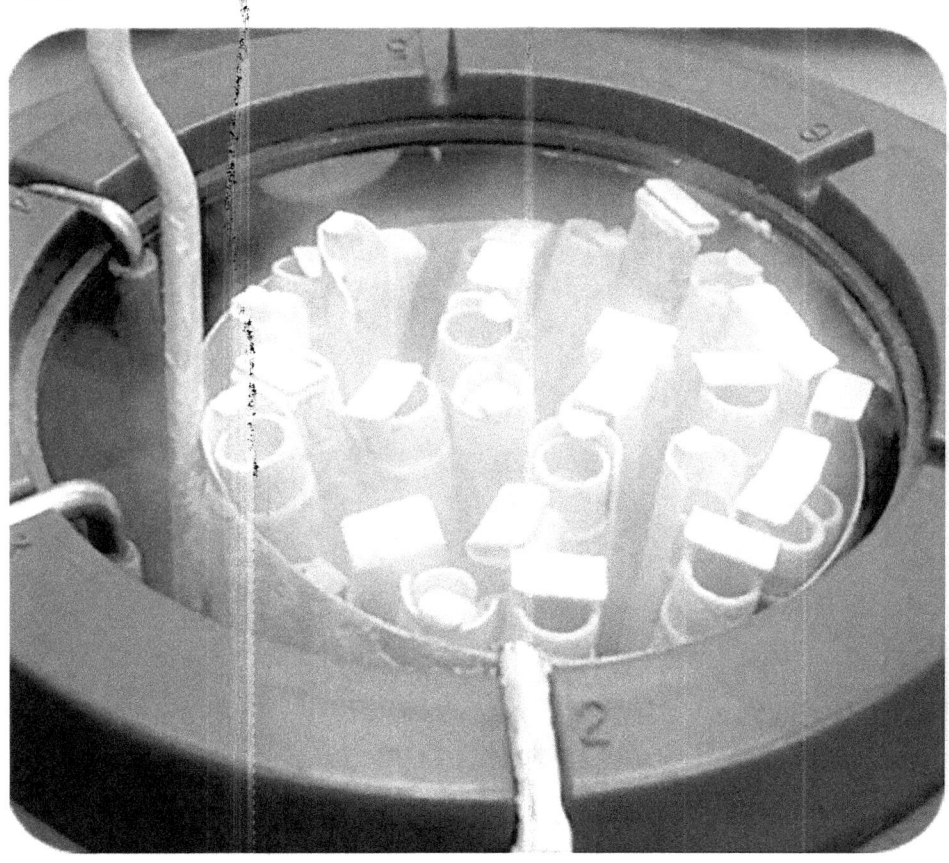

Our Cryogenic Storage

An important aspect to maintain viability of the Umbilical Cord Blood Stem Cells throughout the processing and cryopreservation is controlling the rate of freezing and the subsequent sustained cryogenic temperature of the cells once they are in cryogenic storage.

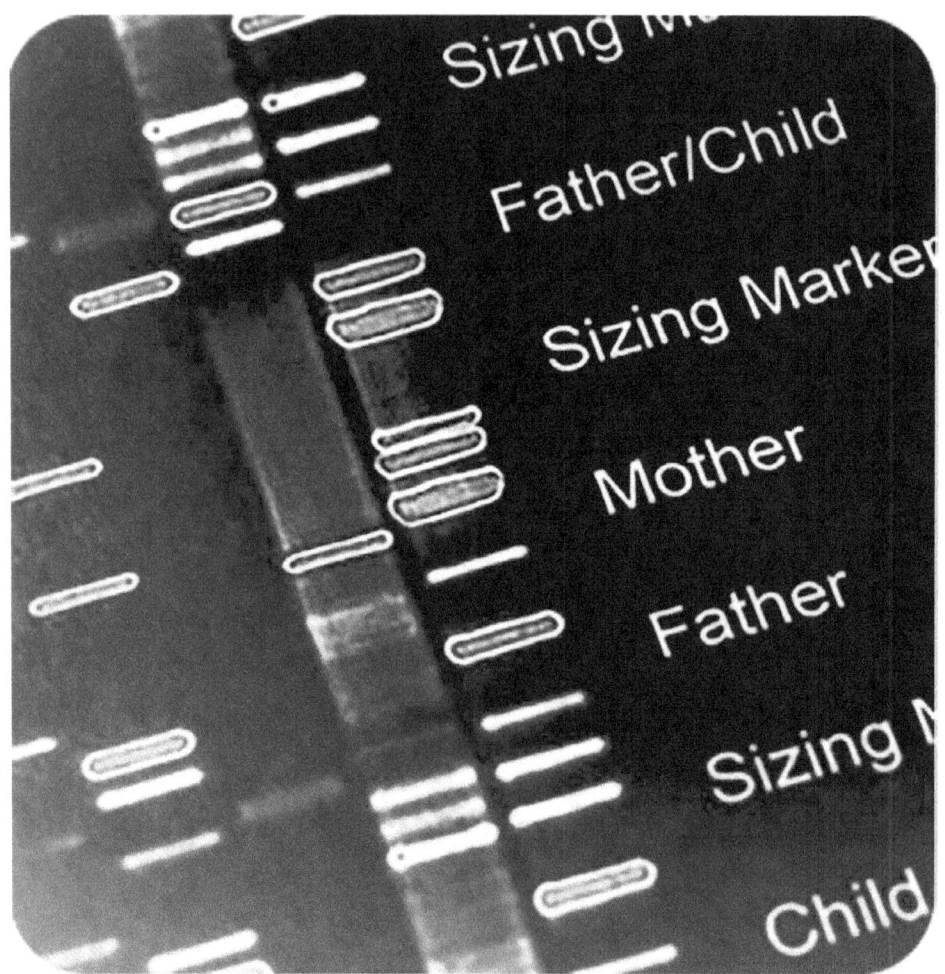

Our laboratory uses a staged freezing process that ensures the cell's future viability. Once the cells are brought to the optimum temperature, they are placed in an overwrap bag and placed in a cryogenic storage cartridge, which then goes into the cryogenic storage tanks.

STEMCELL Lab is a privately-owned laboratory annexed to a full service Clinical Research Laboratory. The Clinical Research Team houses Reliable Research Laboratory.

Our team of scientists has been working together for over 25 years servicing public health facilities, clinical primary care sites of all sizes, hospitals and the pharmaceutical industry.

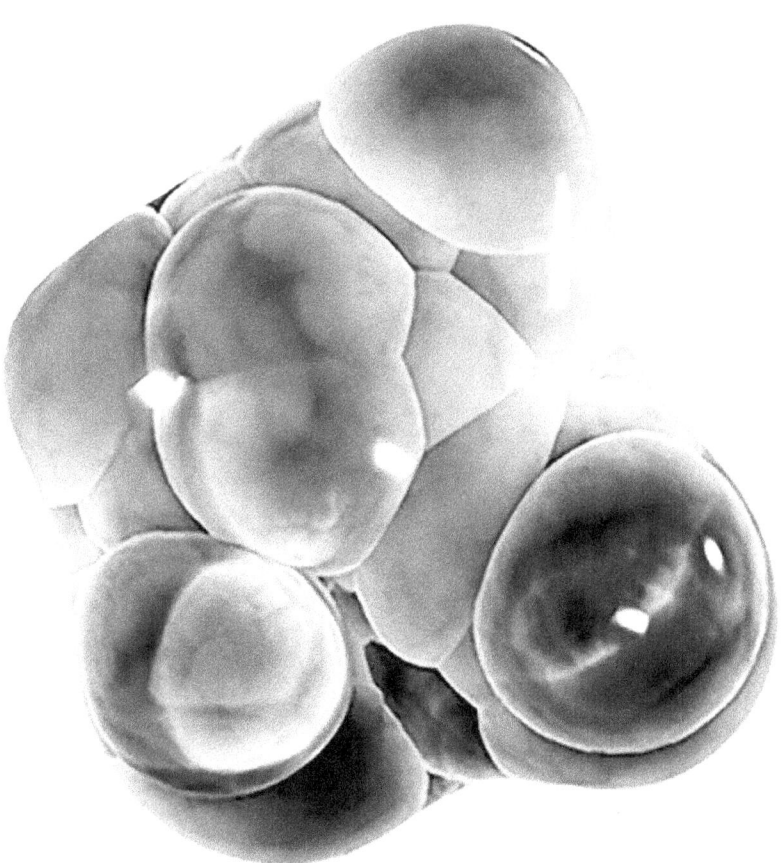

We have completed over 700 research trials catering to the requests of almost every major pharmaceutical company. Our expertise is in partnering with researchers to develop the actual protocols which will be submitted to the FDA for approval. Specifically our focus is in the Clinical Laboratory setting. Our laboratory is currently conducting trials to ascertain the safety and clinical correlation of a wide of array of chemical compounds that will in the end be used to enhance the quality of health care.

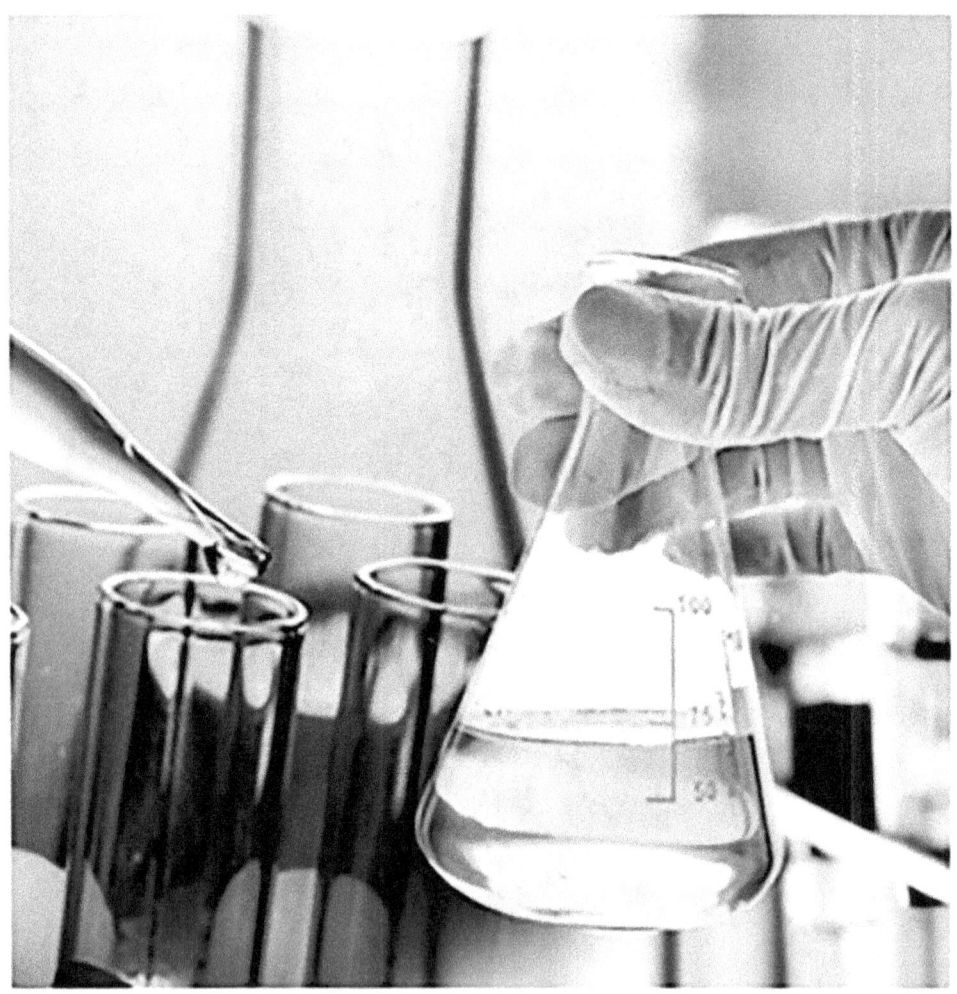

Our Medical Director, Dr. Hugo Romeu , first became interested in Stem Cell Research in 2012 during a trip to Israel. During this visit he met with many prominent young scientists involved in unique experimental incubator groups. The experiments ranged from maintaining extended viability of harvested stem cell products, to extracting human dna and injecting into plants in order to harvest a unique stem cell.

Our mission is to make the harvesting, storage and utilization of stem cells a safe and reliable option to all those in need. Our motto is " Always Reliable". Physicians and patients can count on Stem Cell Lab to harvest, preserve, store and safe guard your stem cells.

STEM CELL LAB is a work in progress. We are a lab within a lab . Our infrastructure is built with a sound foundation in Hematology, Blood Banking , Coagulation, Infectious Disease, Toxicology and Immunology. Most stem cell storage sites do not have their own laboratory. Due to loose regulatory vigilance, simply because of the nuance of this industry, many donors are never guaranteed a safe and reliable process.

Our team handles blood on a daily basis. We are experts in processing, shipping and storage.
We will be involved from the moment the specimen is harvested, to the time when the specimen needs to be used.

Processing

After your child's cord blood has been collected, it can be immediately shipped to our facility. All the necessary materials needed for processing the cord blood sample will arrive at our laboratory under controlled conditions in order to guarantee the safety and sterility of the unit. We process our client's cord blood using a widely accepted and validated volume reduction system.

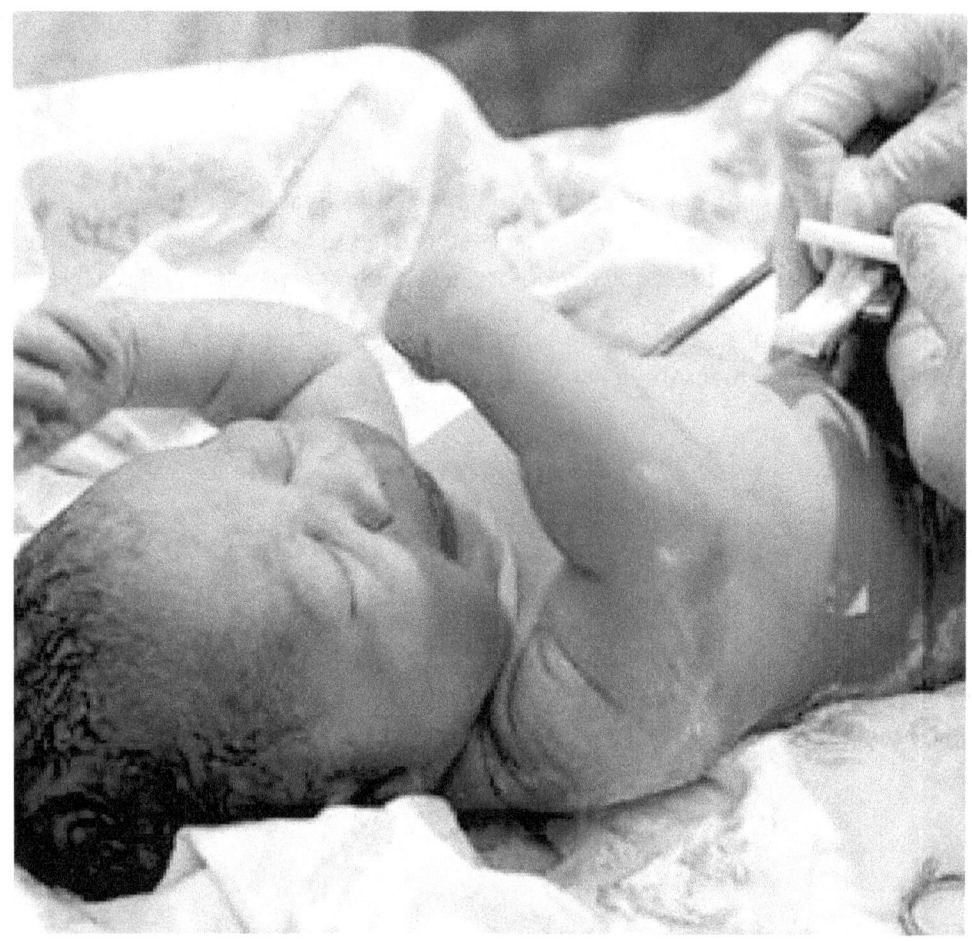

This system is very efficient in recovering a high number of total nucleated cells needed for transplants. As part of our processing procedures we will test the cord blood samples for cell viability and total stem cells using flow cytometry. The cord blood will also be tested to determine the sterility and total nucleated cell count (TNC). The maternal blood collected at the time of delivery will be tested for infectious diseases. All our processing and testing takes place under the strictest quality control conditions.

Storage

To store our clients' invaluable stem cells, we use the best scientifically developed techniques in the area of cryopreservation. First, we use special, compartmentalized cryobags. These bags include two storage chambers one being 20mls, the other 5ml (which could potentially be retained for stem cell expansion once this technology is developed). In addition the cryobags have 2 separate integrally attached segments for testing purposes i.e. HLA-typing. Then, a controlled-rate freezing process is used to prepare the cells for long-term storage. This technique is very important for maintaining the viability of the umbilical cord blood stem cells and for achieving the subsequent and necessary sustained cryogenic temperature in the cryogenic storage. Once the cells are brought to the optimum temperature, they are placed in an Teflon overwrap-bag for added protection and placed in a cryogenic storage cartridge, which then goes into the cryogenic storage tanks. Once the stem cells are properly and safely stored, you, the parent, as the child's guardian, have control over their use and disposal. No stem cells can be released without the parent's consent until the child reaches legal age, in which case control over the stem cells passes to him or her. Based on current research, stem cells can be successfully stored for 25 years in a cryogenic storage. Although not enough years have passed to assert the maximum length of time viable stem cells can be stored with certainty, bone marrow, another similar source of blood cells, has been successfully stored for decades and has remained viable throughout that time.

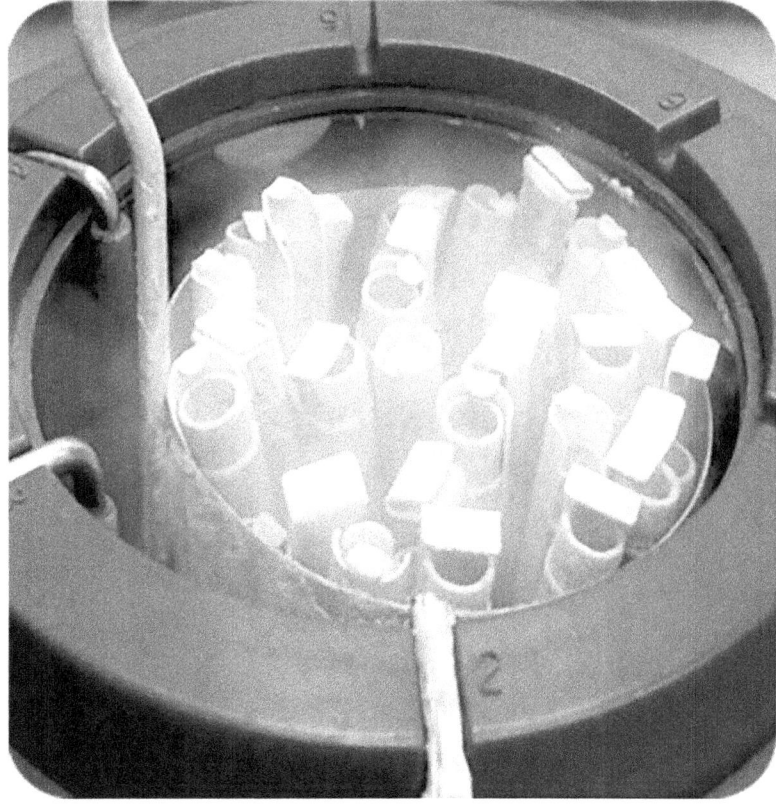

Always at the forefront of stem cell research, processing and cryopreservation, GeneCell International is also one of the few adipose tissue stem cell banks in the world.

Adipose (fat) tissue is a dynamic multi-functional tissue that is found throughout the human body. The stem cells originated from adipose tissue are mesenchymal stem cells which have the ability to differentiate into bone, muscle, fat, nerve, and cartilage. Preliminary research performed at GeneCell International has shown the presence of early stem cells markers as well.

Adipose-derived stem cells are easy to obtain through a simple and localized liposuction process using local anesthesia and with minimal patient discomfort. These autologous adult stem cells show the same morphology, immune phenotype and differentiation capacity as stem cells obtained from bone marrow and umbilical cord blood. They are free of ethical debate and use tissue which is abundant and easy to access. A single sample of adipose tissue can yield more than 200 million stem cells of which 95% are mesenchymal stem cells. These cells appear to be one of the body's tools for self-repair.

Mesenchymal stem cells are capable of performing three important functions with unique abilities:

Plasticity: their potential to transform into other cell types.

Honing: they can travel to the damaged tissue.

Engraftment: their capability to attach themselves to the damaged tissue

Adipose-derived stem cells have the potential to treat a variety of different diseases and conditions that range from breast soft tissue reconstruction after tumor surgery to treatment of brain injuries, stroke, heart failure and more.

Currently, there are several clinical trials using adipose stem cells to treat a variety of disorders, including:

Traumatic Calvaria (skull-cap) Defects

Lipodystrophy I

Myocardial Infarction

Diabetes Type I

Diabetes Type II

Liver Cirrhosis

Maxillary Reconstruction

Chron's Disease

Stem Cell Research and Development

This is being written now

What are stem cells?

Stem Cells are the building blocks of life. They have the unique ability to differentiate into other cell types, and therefore can rebuild organs, tissue, blood systems, and the immune system. Stem cell transplants are used to treat people whose stem cells have been damaged by disease or the treatment of a disease, or as a way to have the donor's immune system fight a blood disorder such as leukemia. Patients requiring a stem cell transplant can access stem cells from three sources: umbilical cord blood, bone marrow, and peripheral blood (blood circulating throughout the body). Stem cells from bone marrow and peripheral blood exist in all healthy adults, but stem cells from these locations are more difficult to match for a transplant patient. Cord blood stem cells, which are harvested and stored at birth, are much easier to match because the immune cells are not developed. Stem cells are at the forefront of one of the most fascinating and revolutionary areas of biology today, and scientists are constantly discovering new uses for them. They hold the potential of allowing researchers to grow and rejuvenate specific cells or tissues, which may ultimately be used to treat major diseases like heart disease, stroke, and Alzheimer's.

Where do you get the stem cells?

Actually human umbilical cord blood is the richest and most viable source of the high quality stem cell. What is Cord Blood? Share More Cord Blood contains stem cells that can save lives The blood left in the umbilical cord after the baby is born, and after the cord is cut, is called cord blood. Cord blood is unique in that it offers a controversy-free way of obtaining stem cells that is quick and painless.

More importantly, these stem cells can reconstitute an immune system, and have the ability to treat, repair, and/or replace damaged cells in the body. Cord blood is abundant in Hematopoietic Stem Cells (HSCs), which are blood-forming stem cells, similar to those contained within bone marrow. Cord blood offers a number of advantages over bone marrow for donors and transplant recipients. It is much easier to collect, often more likely to provide a suitable match than bone marrow stem cells, and stored frozen so it is ready to use. Whereas a bone marrow transplant requires a patient-donor match of 6 out of 6 (or 100%), studies find that cord blood transplants are just as successful with a patient-donor match of 4 out of 6 (or 67%). Cord blood stem cells are currently used to treat patients with immune system and blood diseases including leukemia and lymphoma. Cord Blood Facts Likelihood of an Exact or Partial Match with a Family Member: Match for Donor/Child = 100% Exact Match for Sibling = 25% Exact, 50% Partial Match for Parent = 50% Partial

Why bank stem cells, is it worth the price and effort?

It's like an insurance policy, a safety net, an unexpected opportunity. Science is constantly crossing new frontiers. The latest is the use of stem cells for almost any disease you can think of. Imagine a cell that can merge with your own current cells in your body, and accelerate the healing process Cord blood banking is the simple process of safely and securely storing the blood within your child's umbilical cord, as well as the tissue from the cord itself. A life-giving opportunity that happens only at the time of a birth, it offers a powerful medical resource in fighting devastating chronic and acute diseases. Banking your baby's stem cells offers a unique opportunity to provide protection and security for your family. By choosing to bank your baby's cord blood and tissue with NECBB, you will preserve your family's chance to potentially use it as a part of a treatment therapy for over eighty diseases, including various cancers, genetic diseases, blood disorders, and immune system deficiencies.

Here are a few key reasons why so many parents are now choosing to bank their child's cord blood and cord tissue: ◦Saving these stem cells offers the potential to save your baby's or another family member's life ◦Banking is a once-in-a-

lifetime opportunity available immediately after birth ◦The cord blood and cord tissue collection process is simple and painless to the baby and mother ◦30%-70% of people who need bone marrow transplants cannot find a match, whereas banking your baby's stem cells improves the odds of having a proper match for your baby or another family member ◦Medical advances are allowing stem cells to treat even more diseases and be used in more transplant cases than current medical practices Treatment with Cord Blood Stem Cells Stem cells are at the forefront of one of the most fascinating and revolutionary areas of biology today. Doctors recognize that stem cells can help treat numerous diseases by generating healthy new cells and tissue.

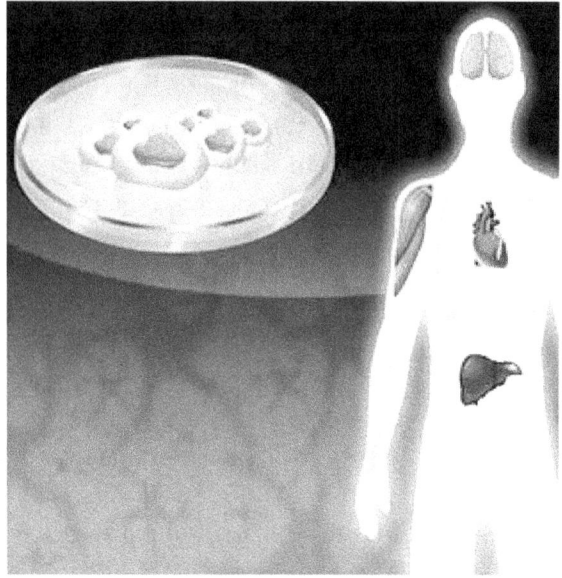

There are a wide range of diseases that are treatable with cord blood, including stem cell disorders, acute and chronic forms of leukemia, myeloproliferative disorders, and many more. In addition to the host of conditions that can now be treated, it's the potential of cord blood that holds the most excitement as research continues to uncover new possibilities. The efficacy of treating disease with cord blood stem cells is real. Beyond their potential to grow and rejuvenate specific cells or tissues, which can ultimately be used to treat a host of diseases, cord blood stem cells are currently being used to treat more than eighty acute and chronic diseases today. Diseases That Can be Treated by Stem Cell Transplantation: ◦Stem Cell Disorders ◦Aplastic Anemia (Severe) ◦Fanconi Anemia ◦Paroxysmal Nocturnal Hemoglobinuria (PNH) ◦Acute Leukemias ◦Acute Lymphoblastic Leukemia (ALL) ◦Acute Myelogenous Leukemia (AML) ◦Acute Biphenotypic Leukemia ◦Acute Undifferentiated Leukemia ◦Chronic Leukemias ◦Chronic Myelogenous Leukemia (CML) ◦Chronic Lymphocytic Leukemia (CLL) ◦Juvenile Chronic Myelogenous Leukemia (JCML) ◦Juvenile Myelomonocytic Leukemia (JMML) ◦Myeloproliferative Disorders ◦Acute Myelofibrosis ◦Agnogenic Myeloid Metaplasia (myelofibrosis) ◦Polycythemia Vera ◦Essential Thrombocythemia ◦Myelodysplastic Syndromes ◦Refractory Anemia (RA) ◦Refractory Anemia with Ringed Sideroblasts (RARS) ◦Refractory Anemia with Excess Blasts (RAEB) ◦Refractory Anemia with Excess Blasts in Transformation (RAEB-T) ◦Chronic Myelomonocytic Leukemia (CMML) ◦Lymphoproliferative Disorders ◦Non-Hodgkin's Lymphoma ◦Hodgkin's Disease ◦Prolymphocytic Leukemia ◦Inherited Erythrocyte Abnormalities ◦Beta Thalassemia Major ◦Pure Red Cell Aplasia ◦Sickle Cell Disease ◦Cartilage-Hair Hypoplasia ◦Glanzmann Thrombasthenia ◦Osteopetrosis ◦Other Malignancies ◦Breast Cancer ◦Ewing Sarcoma ◦Neuroblastoma ◦Renal Cell Carcinoma ◦Waldenstrom's Macroglobulinemia ◦Other Inherited Disorders ◦Lesch-Nyhan Syndrome ◦Liposomal Storage Diseases ◦Mucopolysaccharidoses (MPS) ◦Hurler Syndrome (MPS-IH) ◦Scheie Syndrome (MPS-IS) ◦Hunter's Syndrome (MPS-II) ◦Sanfilippo Syndrome (MPS-III) ◦Morquio Syndrome (MPS-IV) ◦Maroteaux-Lamy Syndrome (MPS-VI) ◦Sly Syndrome, Beta-Glucuronidase Deficiency (MPS-VII) ◦Adrenoleukodystrophy ◦Mucolipidosis II (I-cell Disease) ◦Krabbe Disease ◦Gaucher's Disease ◦Niemann-Pick Disease ◦Wolman Disease ◦Metachromatic Leukodystrophy ◦Histiocytic Disorders ◦Familial Erythrophagocytic Lymphohistiocytosis ◦Histiocytosis-X ◦Hemophagocytosis ◦Phagocyte Disorders ◦Chediak-Higashi Syndrome ◦Chronic Granulomatous Disease ◦Neutrophil Actin Deficiency ◦Reticular Dysgenesis ◦Congenital Immune System Disorders ◦Ataxia-Telangiectasia ◦Kostmann Syndrome ◦Leukocyte Adhesion Deficiency ◦DiGeorge Syndrome ◦Bare Lymphocyte Syndrome ◦Omenn's Syndrome ◦Severe Combined Immunodeficiency (SCID) ◦SCID with Adenosine Deaminase Deficiency ◦Absence of T & B Cells SCID ◦Absence of T Cells, Normal B Cell SCID ◦Common Variable Immunodeficiency ◦Wiskott-Aldrich Syndrome ◦X-Linked Lymphoproliferative Disorder ◦Inherited Platelet Abnormalities ◦Amegakaryocytosis / Congenital Thrombocytopenia ◦Plasma Cell Disorders ◦Multiple Myeloma.

Romeu Clinical Enterprises
Dr. Hugo Romeu M.D.

ROMEU CLINICAL
ENTERPRISES

dr.hugoromeu@yahoo.com

Romeu Clinical Enterprises

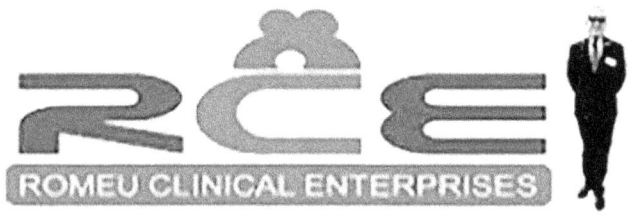

ROMEU CLINICAL

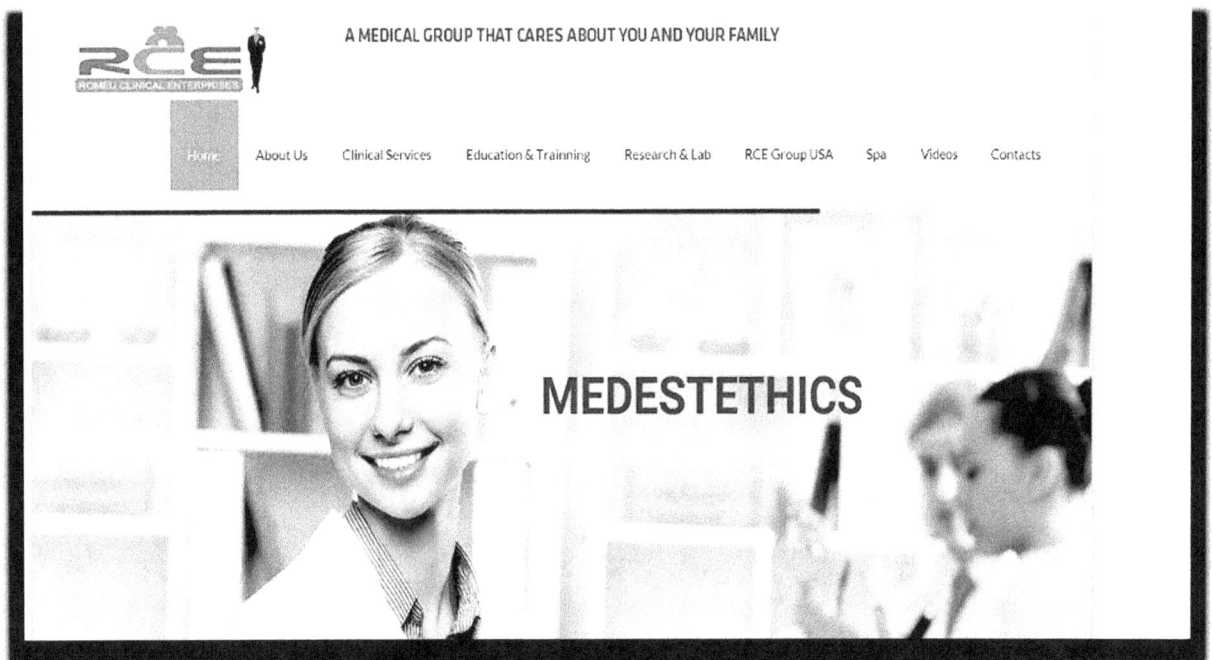

Romeu Clinical Medical offers a variety of services and link with Posgraduated Study Programs, Reserch studies, and more.

Romeu Clinical Spa

Romeu Clinical Medical Spa offers a variety of cosmetic medical aesthetics services and cosmetic surgical services to rejuvenate your appearance in a comfortable, state-of-the-art cosmetic surgery facility.

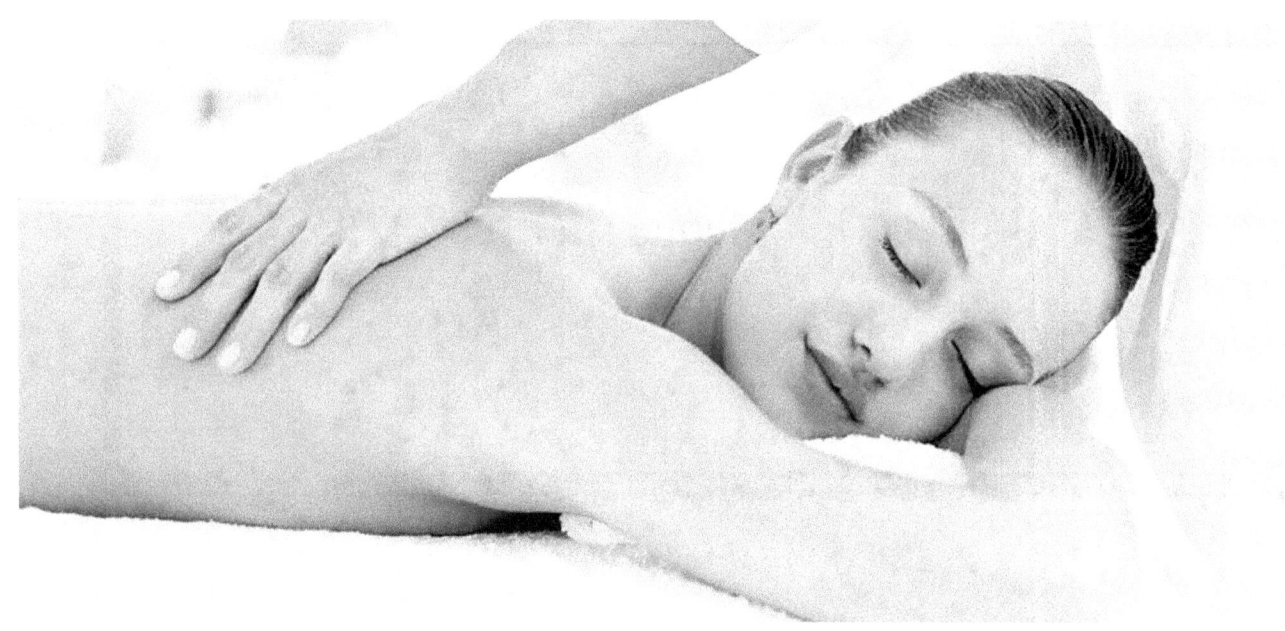

Qualified Doctors

We are fully accredited for office based surgery by the Joint Commission, and we are pleased to provide you with state-of-the-art medical and surgical aesthetics.

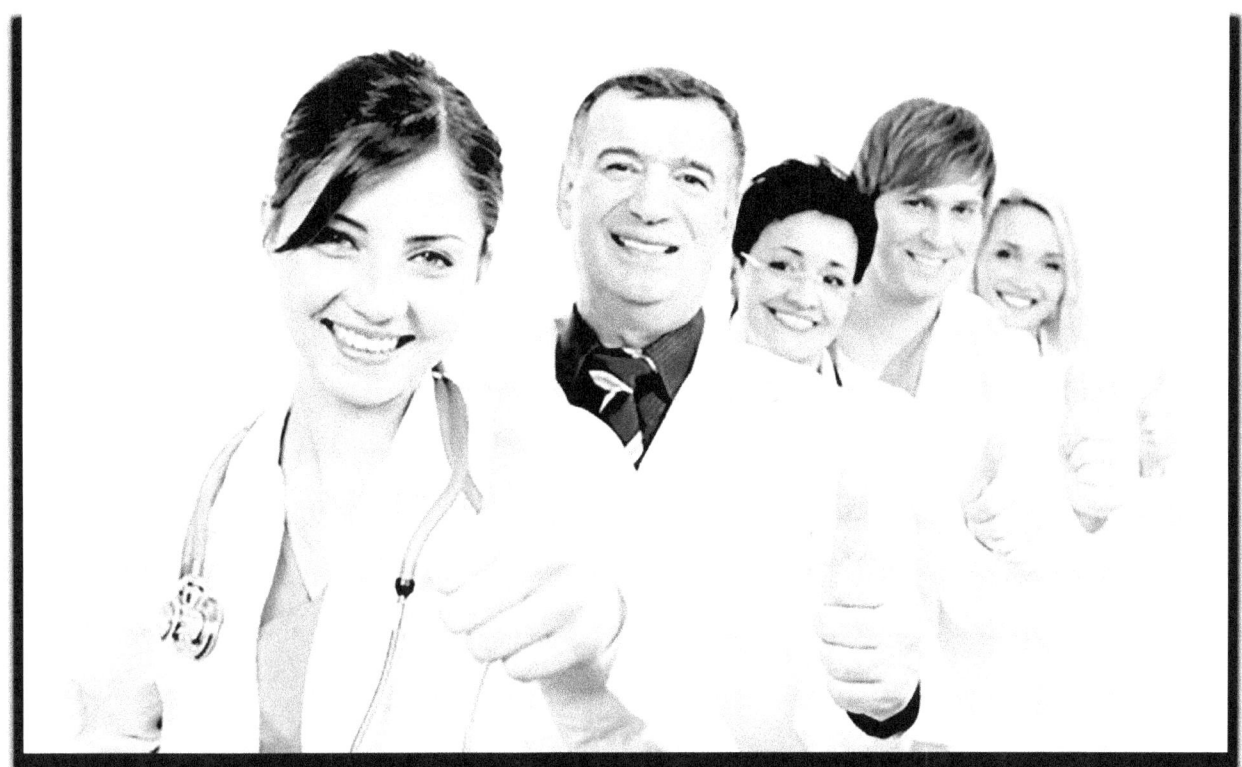

Technology

At Romeu Clinical Medical Medical Spa, we use state-of-the-art, computerized aesthetic photo analysis including Beau Visage, which detects and maps melanin, blood, and sun damage in the skin, and Physiometrics.

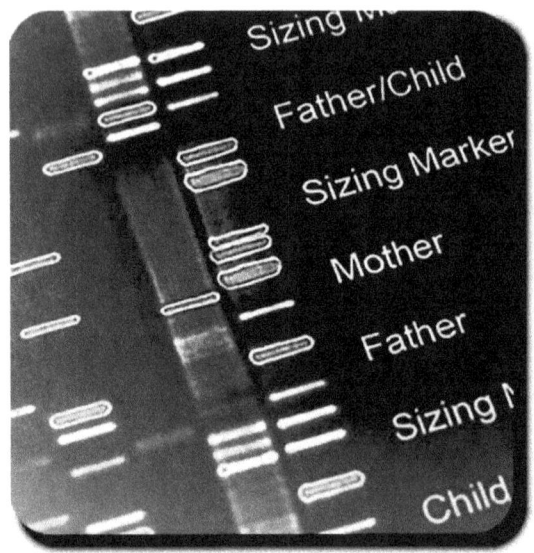

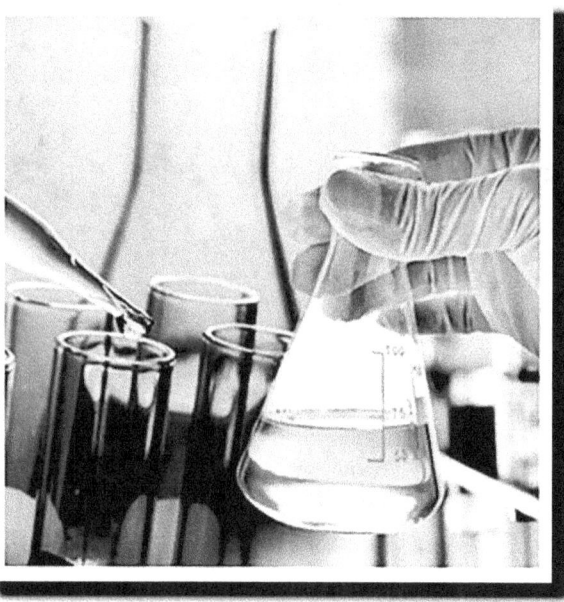

Our Philosophy

In 1995 Romeu Clinical Enterprises was formed to provide diversified services for other physicians. The company was created by Dr. Hugo Romeu to combine a wide array of consultant based deliverables to other health care providers, both individuals and companies.

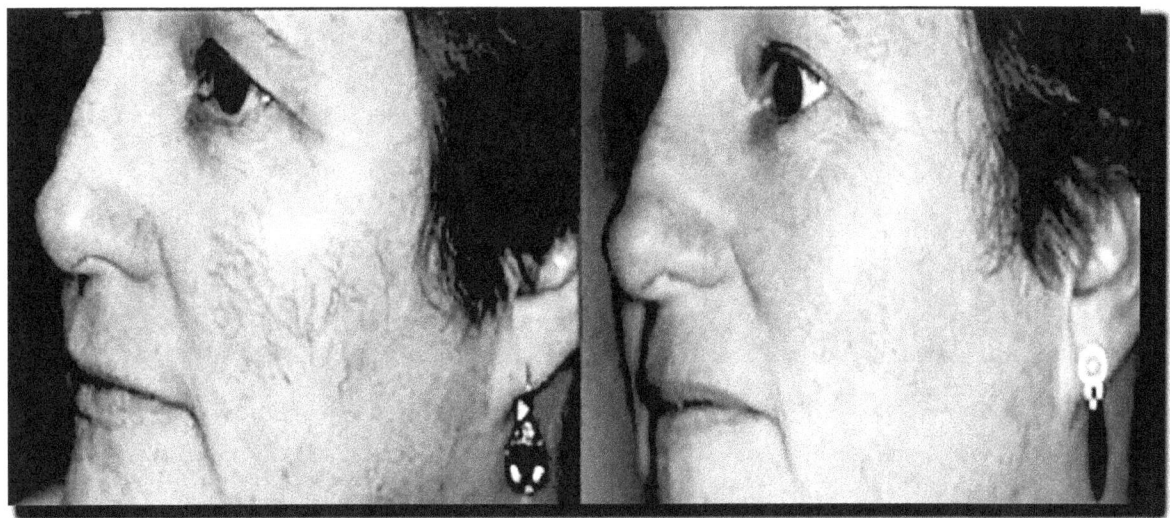

The concept originated from the prior job from 1984- 1994: which included positions in government based laboratories, medical examiners offices to the direction of a series of large clinical laboratories in Europe, U.S. and the Caribbean.

In the early 90's Romeu began projects in primary health care providing vaccinations, drug screening, immigration profiles and general primary care; to lower socioeconomic cliental. Later he developed skin care along with spa related health services for an altogether different population.

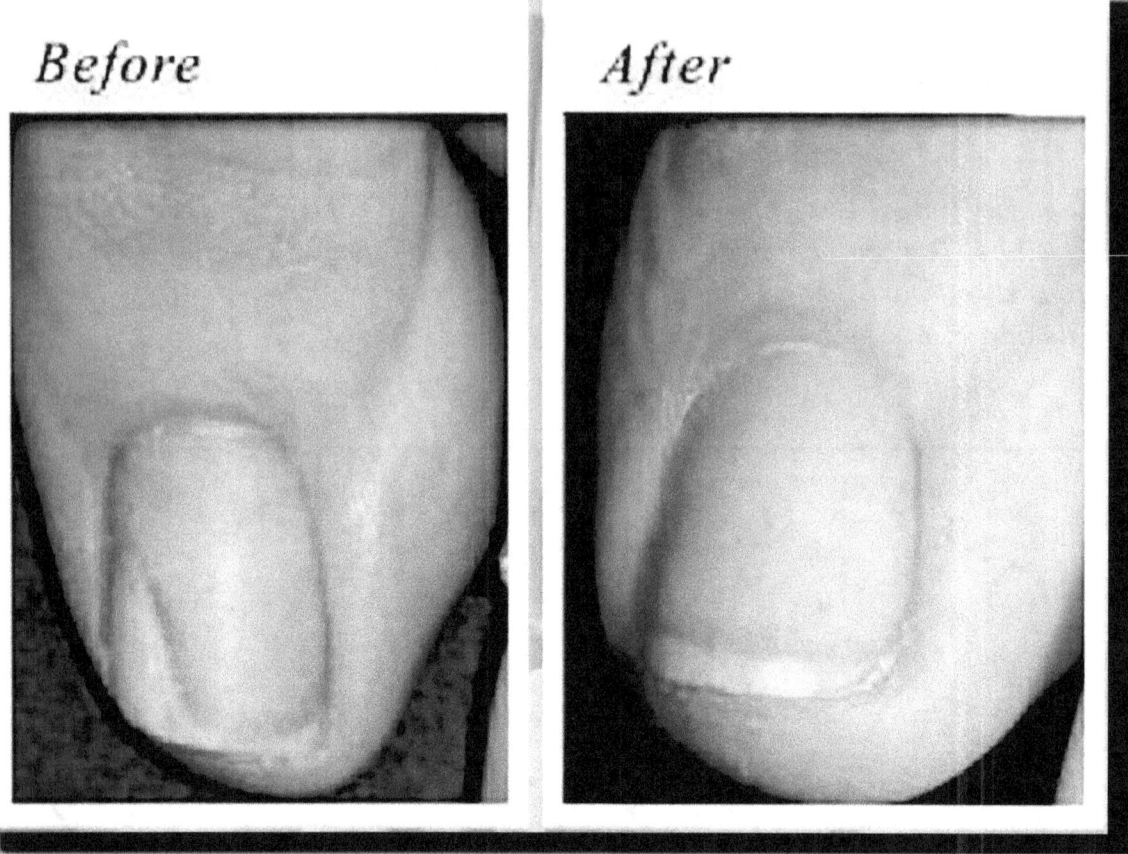

Before   **After**

The culmination of experiences resulted in the formation of a RCE Group USA, with a focus on over all wellness, preventative care and most important education and training.

We recently re organized the company to focus on Research, Clinical Laboratory, and Education. The spa related components are provided by ancillary affiliations with Derm Spa and Prestige Laser Hair removal.

Romeu Clinical Medical Spa offers a variety of cosmetic medical aesthetics services and cosmetic surgical services to rejuvenate your appearance in a comfortable, state-of-the-art cosmetic surgery facility.

Treatments

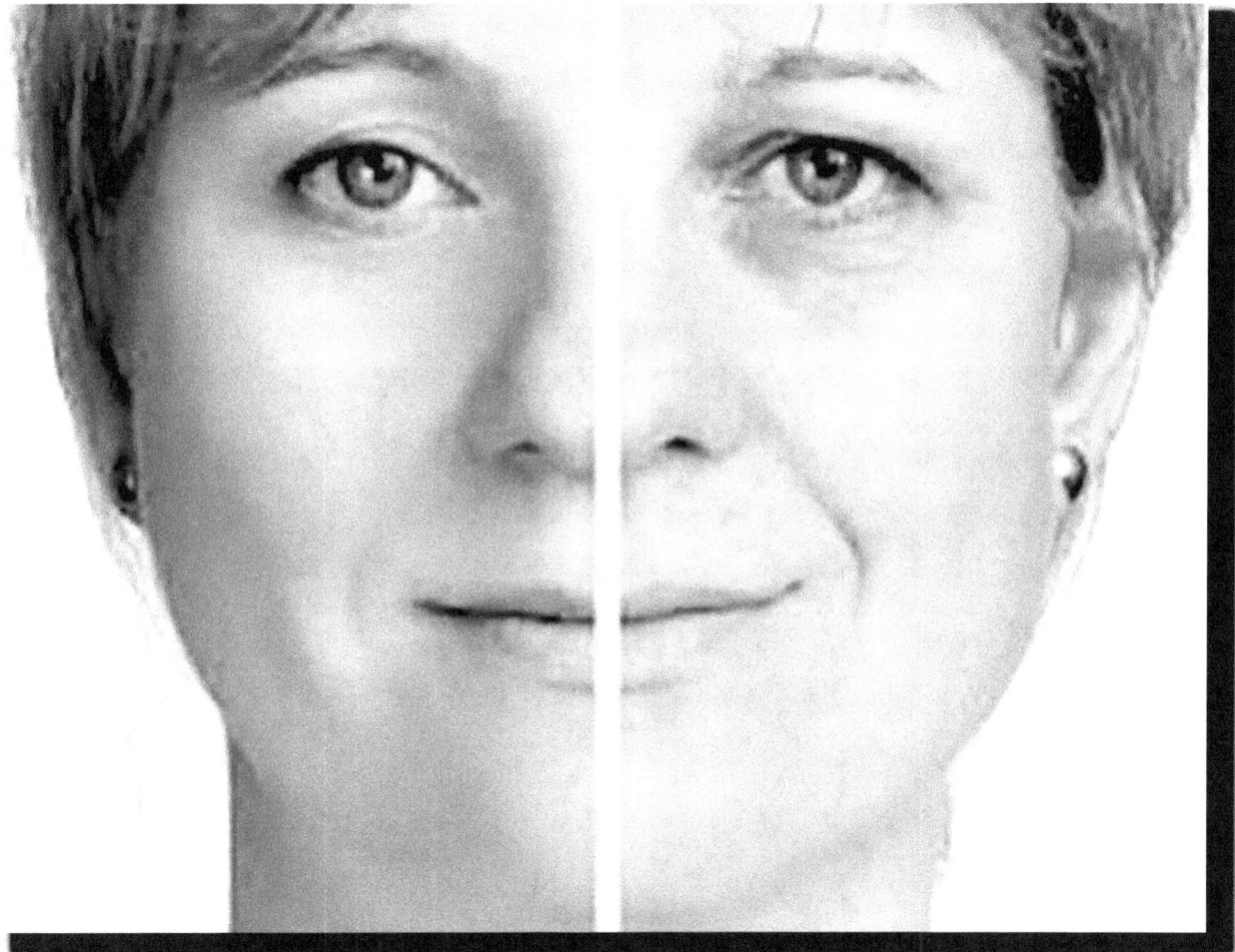

We constantly work to give you not only a professional and results focused service but also a pampering and stress relieving experience – all set within a relaxing, peaceful and friendly atmosphere.

Skin treatments

We offer: *Anti-Ageing Treatments, including Skin Rejuvenation and Wrinkle Relaxing Treatments. *Skin Treatments.

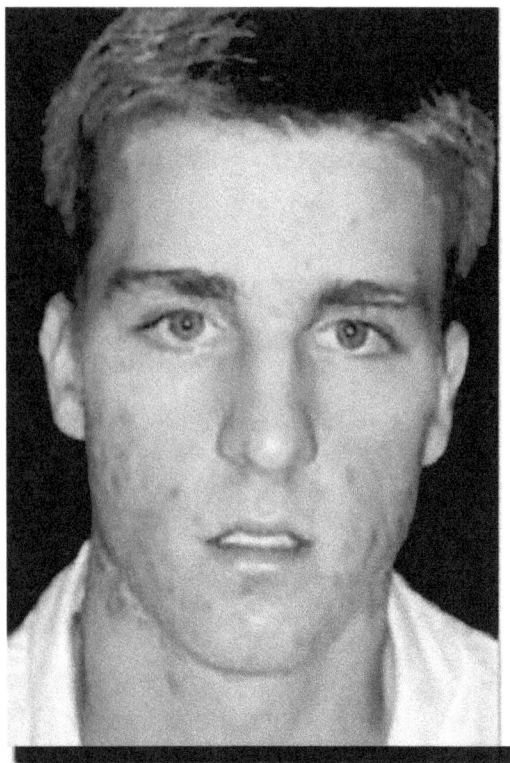 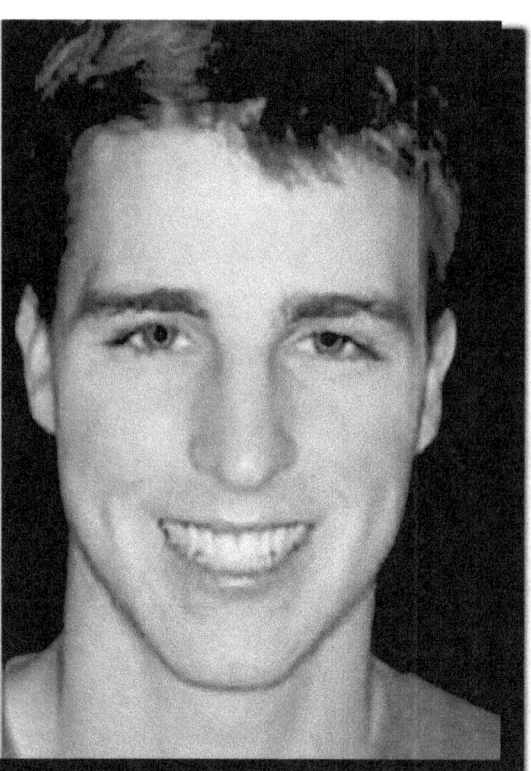

<u>Burn Fat & Reshape your Body</u>

Believe in the possibility of lasting change. You deserve to take some time just for you, your health and well-being.

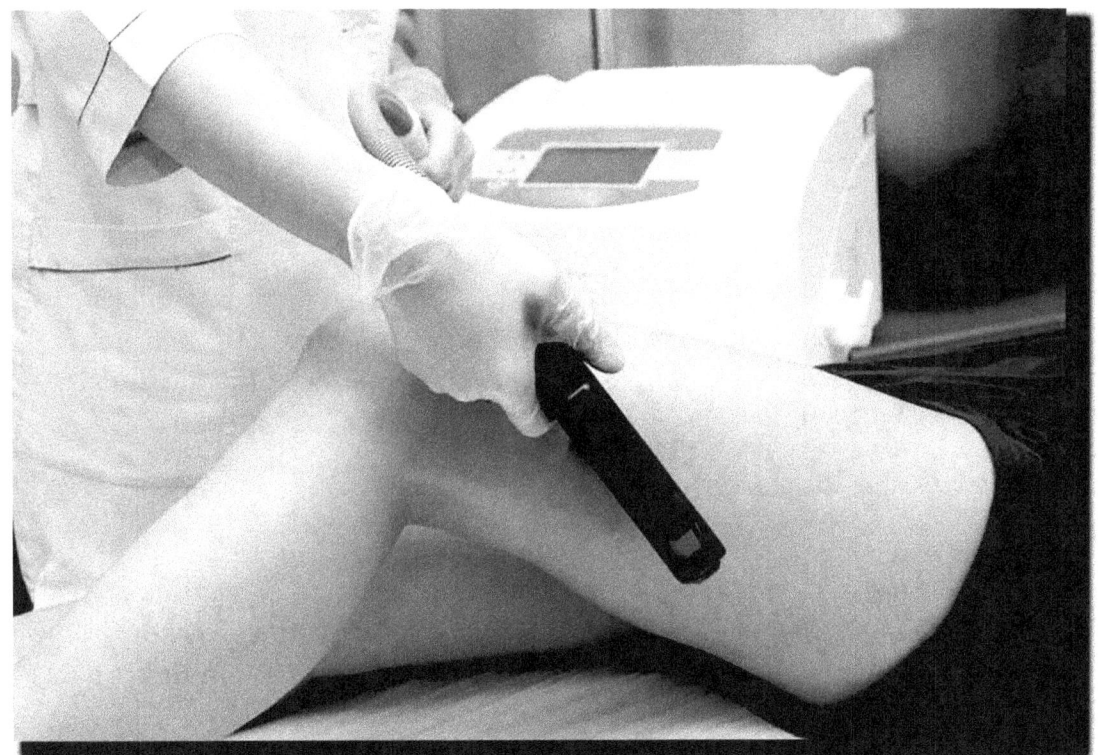

Unwanted Hair Removed (Women, Men and Teens)

Unwanted hair is a common problem for both women and men. Many of us wish that we did not have to shave, wax, use depilatory creams or resort to any other temporary hair removal methods ever again. Thanks to advances in Laser Hair Removal technology, now you can enjoy a clean hair-free body and throw away your inventory of razors, waxes and creams.

At Studio Esthetique, our friendly and experienced staff will help you achieve your goal of a hair-free body. We use the latest, FDA approved, Laser Hair Removal equipment (including Alexandrite and Nd: YAG lasers) that allows us to custom-tailor the treatments for individuals with all skin and hair types.

How Does Laser Hair Removal Work?

Lasers produce a beam of highly concentrated light that is absorbed by the melanin, or pigment, located in hair follicles. Light is converted to heat, causing thermal damage to hair follicles without harming the surrounding skin. The heat has a disabling effect on numerous hair follicles at once and results in the gradual reduction of hair re-growth.

Am I a Candidate For Laser Hair Removal?

If you are concerned about unwanted hair for cosmetic or medical reasons, tired of temporary hair removal methods, or experience a problem with ingrown hairs, you are a candidate for laser hair removal. Schedule a Free Consultation today and get professional advice.

What Body Area Can Be Treated?
Lasers can be safely and effectively used to remove hair on any area of the human body.

All stetic treatmens

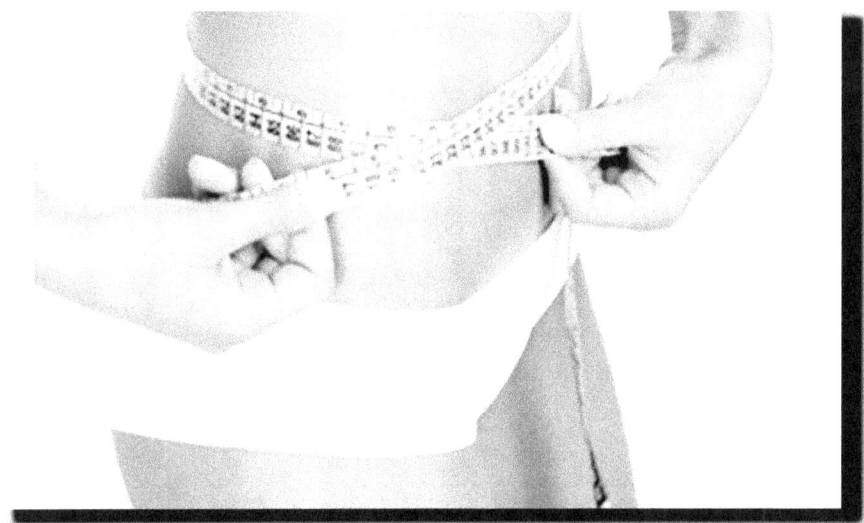

Go to our website and link with all services we offer

www.romeuclinical.com

Beauty & Skin by Dr. Hugo Romeu

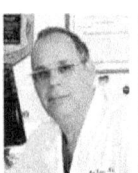

Dr. Hugo Romeu received formal training in experimental laboratory medicine at several prestigious institutions such as Roswell Park Memorial Institute, State University of New York and Cook County Hospital.

He has published, written protocols and participated in study desighns in all phases of research, from pre-clinical animal trials to late phase studies. Over the last 32 years he has completed 672 trials, the majority phase one and bioequivalence. Formally trained in dermatopathology at the State University of New York, his career as an expert is the structure and function of skin has spanned out over 25 years for prestigious institutions across the globe. The doctor has been involved in cutting edge research to identify safety and efficacy of topical skin products for the pharmaceutical and cosmetic industry. Dr. Romeu is known as the " doctors' doctor " in the arena of skin care. To date he has over 300 completed research projects for compounds utilized in the treatment of acne, wrinkles, skin pigmentation and much more. Recently his work has been utilized by leading over the county anti-aging products consumed by an elite population. His base is in Miami, where he owns and operates Reliable Research Laboratory and Romeu Clinical Enterprises.

Scores of books are available on the market which addresses rejuvenation, wrinkles, and general skin issues.

This book is unique because it is written from a scientific foundation, and tempered by a holistic lifestyle.

As a physician use to dealing with the public, to put things in laymen's terms is essential. To provide a simple explanation of complex terms is an art, and that is what makes this book special.

The reader will be left with the basic understanding of the structure and function of the skin. The idea is to offer a solution along with the description of many issues; from acne to wrinkles.

I guarantee you will know more about your skin, and how to improve when finished. Is currently the managing partner and is on board around the clock to make sure that Reliable Research lab maintains the high expectations this industry demands.

Dr. Hugo Romeu M.D.

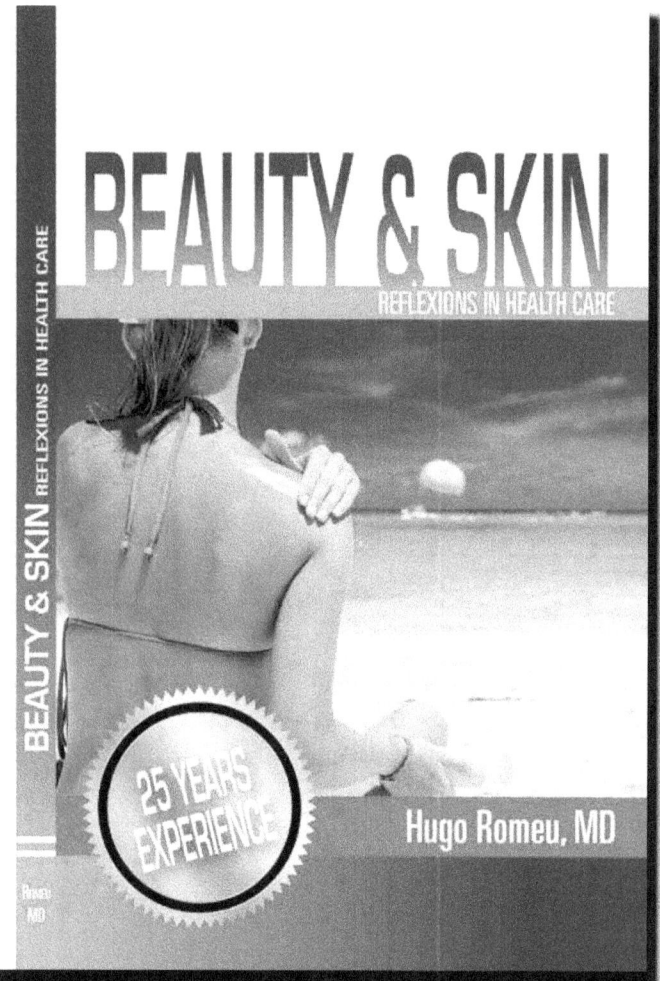

https://www.amazon.com/Beauty-Skin-Reflections-Practical-Approach/dp/1530595495/ref=sr_1_1?s=books&ie=UTF8&qid=1493746100&sr=1-1&keywords=beauty+%26+skin+hugo+romeu

CRI Phase 1
Dr. Hugo Romeu M.D.

CRI PHASE 1

dr.hugoromeu@yahoo.com

CRI Phase 1

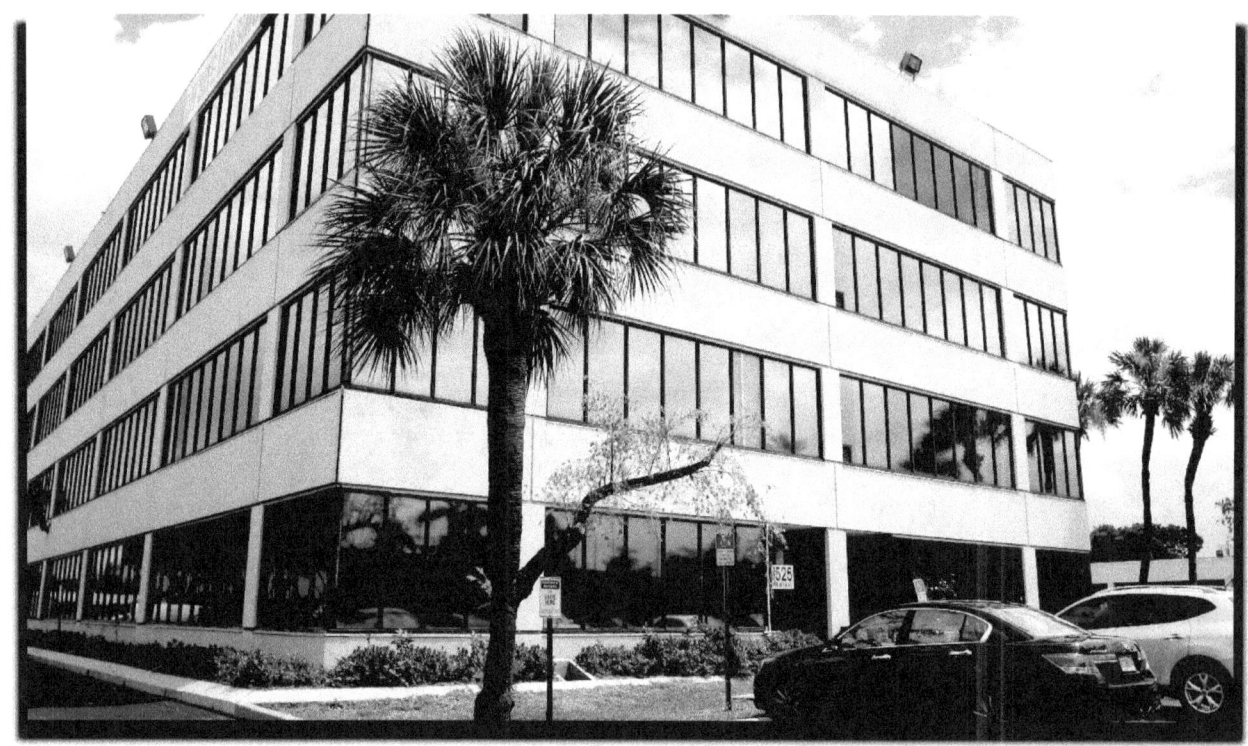

1505 NW 167 St, Suite 200

Miami, Fl 33169

The Clinical Research Institute Phase 1 , is a site where the Principal Investigators and Research Coordinators have extensive experience conducting Phase I-IV Clinical Trials in multiple therapeutic areas like Asthma, COPD, Gout, Hypertension, Osteoarthritis, Rheumatoid Arthritis, Diabetes Mellitus, Hyperlipidemia, Obesity, Liver Cirrhosis, Chronic Renal Insufficiency, Anxiety and Depression Disorder, ADHD, Bipolar Disorder, Insomnia, Chronic Back Pain, Healthy Voluntaries Studies, Parkinson's Disease, Multiple Sclerosis, Woman Health, etc.

Principal Investigators: Dr. Hugo Romeu, MD (Internist, Pathologist), Dr. Michael M. Pfeffer, MD (Neurologist, Internist), Dr. Mario Cuervo (Psychiatry)

Dr. Romeu has been involved in 672 Clinical Laboratory Research Trials over the last 32 years.

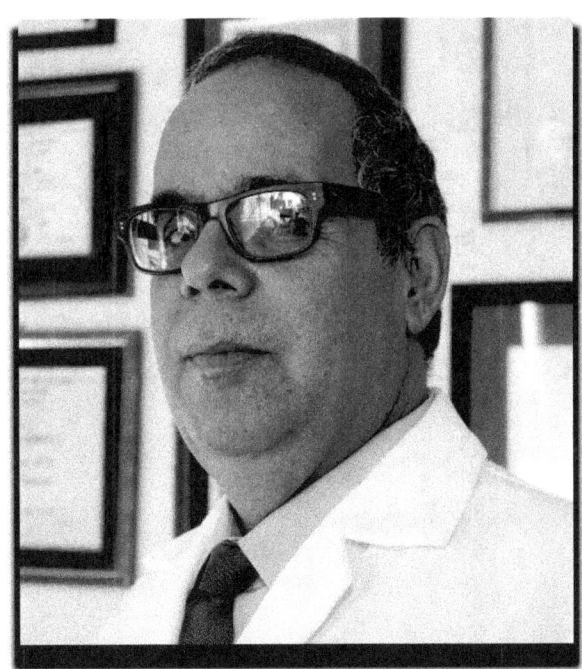

His experience began with formal post graduate training in experimental pathology, at which time he developed protocols for identification of circulating antibodies for early detection of insulin dependence. From pre-clinical trials to late phase projects, he has a lifetime of direct clinical research exposure.

Dr. Romeu has completed studies for all the major Pharmaceutical Laboratories , as well as numerous smaller companies. He can write or develop your protocol, than make sure that any trial is carried out with the highest scientific and ethical standards.

A definite plus is the Dr. Romeu is not only the principal owner , but is also directly involved with the daily operations.

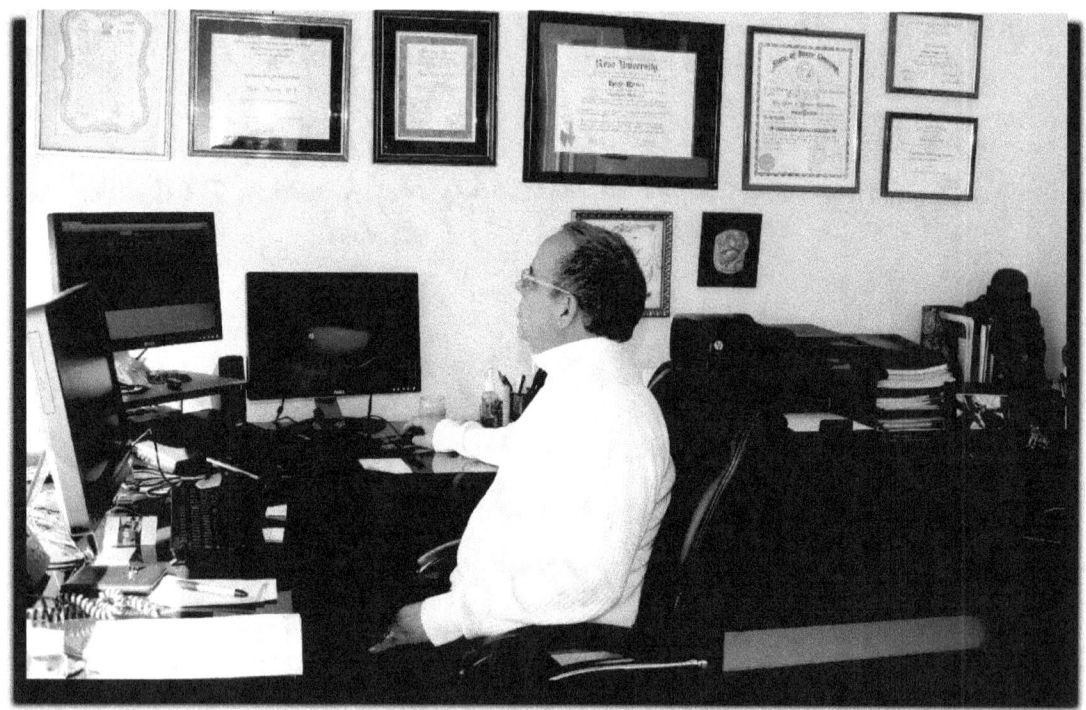

Our site capacities include:

Easy access to expressways connecting East-West and North-South, 35,000 sq ft building, 35 bed capacity, PK area, Temperature Controlled Double Lock Drug Room, Spacious and Equiped Laboratory Area, Refrigerated Centrifuge, -20ᵒC and -70ᵒC Freezers, Lunch and Recreational Patient Area, Nursing Station, Private Examination Rooms, Calibrated ECG Machines, Spirometry Machines, Scales, as well as Manual and Electronic Blood Pressure Machines, Conference Room, Monitor's Rooms, Wireless Internet Access, Coordinators Working Area, Dedicated Business Development Department, Quality Control and Quality Assurance Department, Reception Area, Waiting Area, Car Parking Space, On Site Record Retention Area,

Regulatory Department, Access to Dry Ice, emergency generator and most importantly an extensive database of potential research participants.

Choosing to participate in a clinical trial is an important personal decision. The following frequently asked questions provide detailed information about clinical trials. In addition, it is often helpful to talk to a physician, family members, or friends about deciding to join a trial. After identifying some trial options, the next step is to contact the study research staff and ask questions about specific trials.

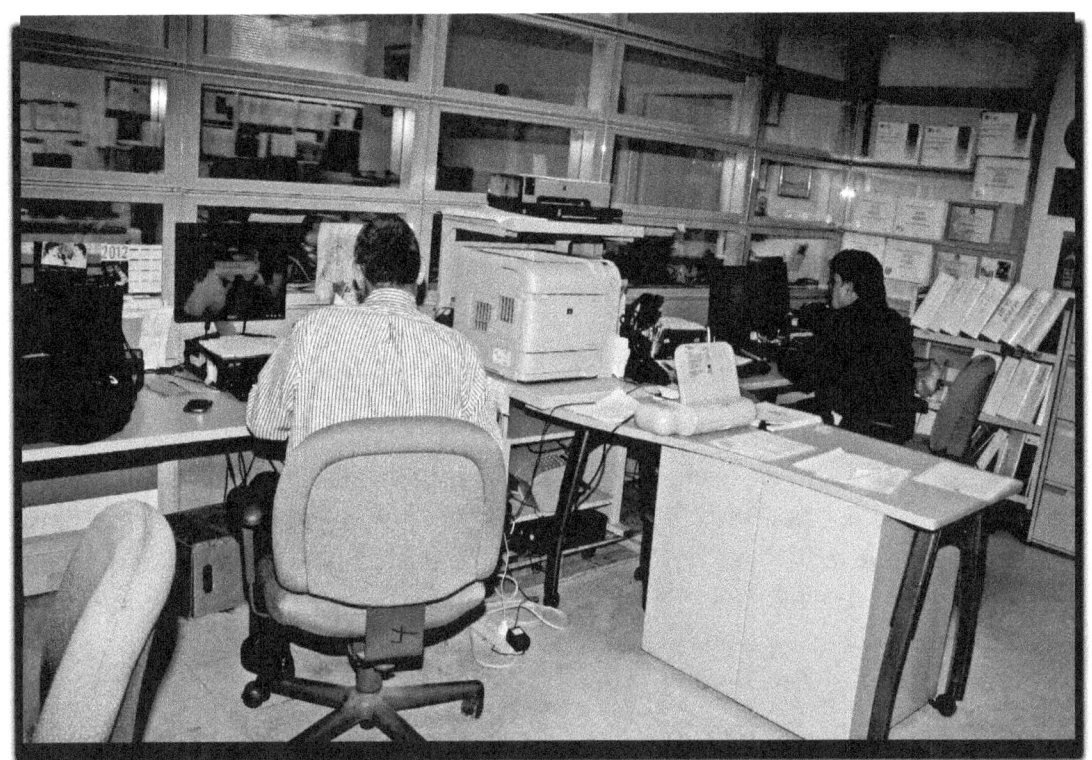

Can a participant leave a clinical trial after it has begun?

Yes. A participant can leave a clinical trial, at any time. When withdrawing from the trial, the participant should let the research team know about it, and the reasons for leaving the study.

Does a participant continue to work with a primary health care provider while in a trial?

Yes. Most clinical trials provide short-term treatments related to a designated illness or condition, but do not provide extended or complete primary health care. In addition, by having the health care provider work with the research team, the participant can ensure that other medications or treatments will not conflict with the protocol.

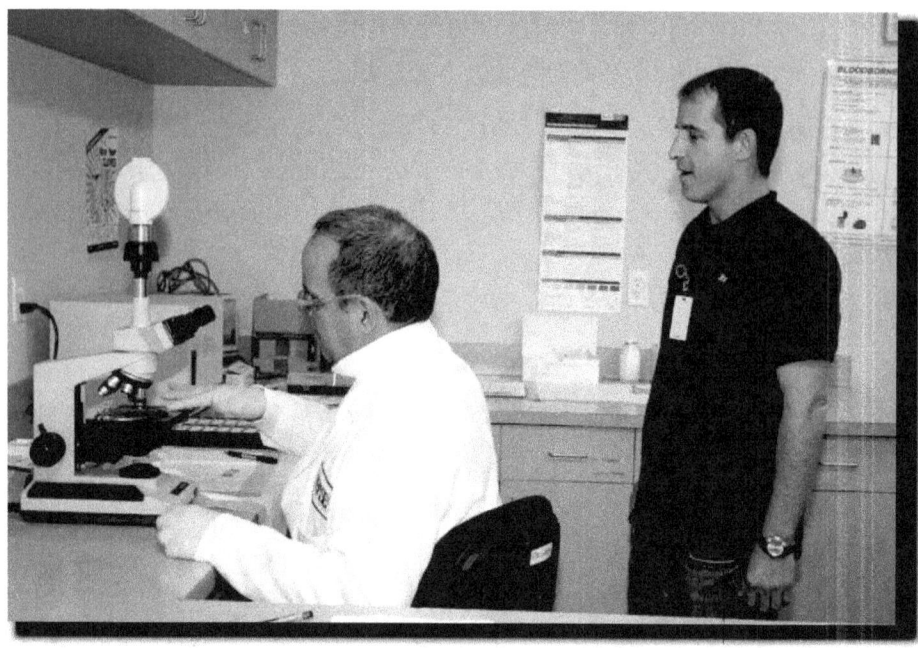

How is the safety of the participant protected?

The ethical and legal codes that govern medical practice also apply to clinical trials. In addition, most clinical research is federally regulated with built in safeguards to protect the participants. The trial follows a carefully controlled protocol, a study plan which details what researchers will do in the study. As a clinical trial progresses, researchers report the results of the trial at scientific meetings, to medical journals, and to various government agencies. Individual participants' names will remain secret and will not be mentioned in these reports.

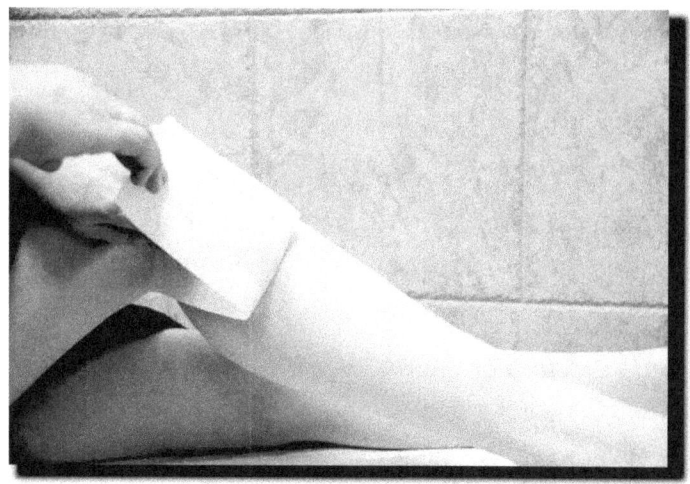

What are side effects and adverse reactions?

Side effects are any undesired actions or effects of the experimental drug or treatment. Negative or adverse effects may include headache, nausea, hair loss, skin irritation, or other physical problems. Experimental treatments must be evaluated for both immediate and long-term side effects.

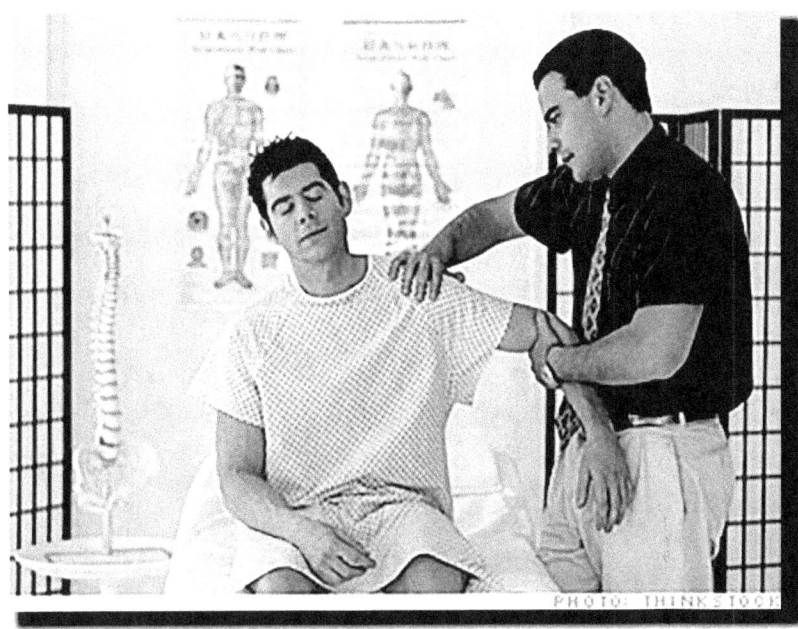

What are the benefits and risks of participating in a clinical trial?

Benefits

Clinical trials that are well-designed and well-executed are the best approach for eligible participants to:

Play an active role in their own health care.

Gain access to new research treatments before they are widely available.

Obtain expert medical care at leading health care facilities during the trial.

Help others by contributing to medical research.

Risks

There are risks to clinical trials.

There may be unpleasant, serious or even life-threatening side effects to experimental treatment.

The experimental treatment may not be effective for the participant.

The protocol may require more of their time and attention than would a non-protocol treatment, including trips to the study site, more treatments, hospital stays or complex dosage requirements.

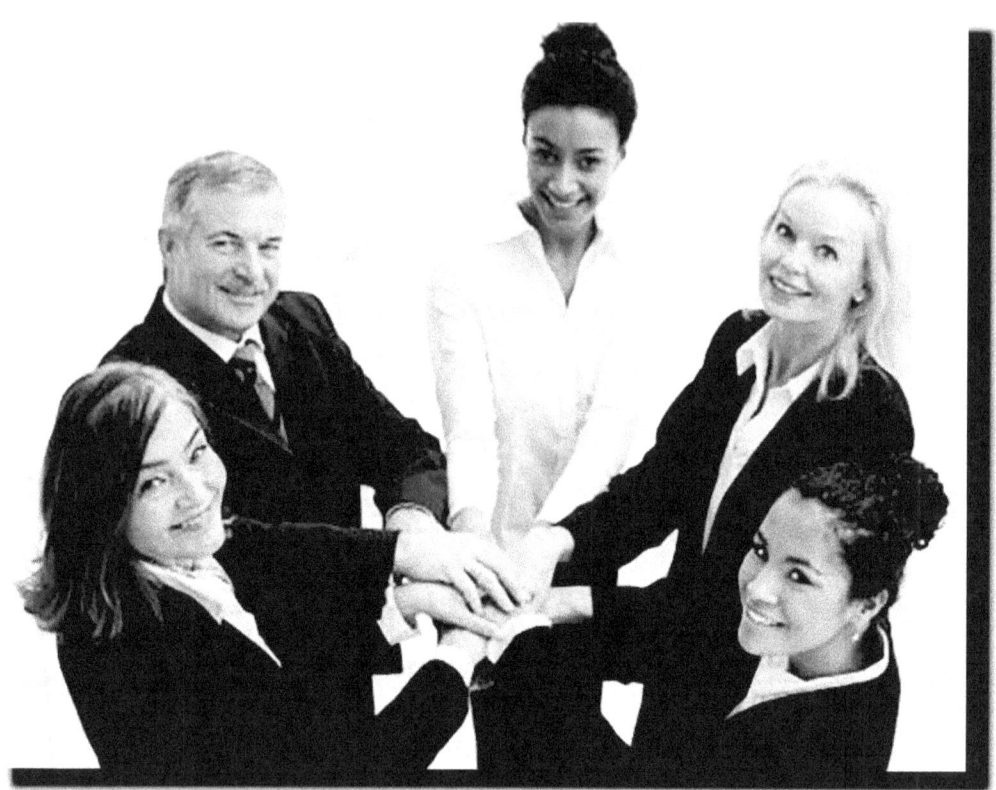

What are the different types of clinical trials?

Treatment trials test experimental treatments, new combinations of drugs, or new approaches to surgery or radiation therapy.

Prevention trials look for better ways to prevent disease in people who have never had the disease or to prevent a disease from returning. These approaches may include medicines, vaccines, vitamins, minerals, or lifestyle changes.

Diagnostic trials are conducted to find better tests or procedures for diagnosing a particular disease or condition.

Screening trials test the best way to detect certain diseases or health conditions.

Quality of Life trials (or Supportive Care trials) explore ways to improve comfort and the quality of life for individuals with a chronic illness.

What are the phases of clinical trials?

Clinical trials are conducted in phases. The trials at each phase have a different purpose and help scientists answer different questions:

In Phase I trials, researchers test an experimental drug or treatment in a small group of people (20-80) for the first time to evaluate its safety, determine a safe dosage range, and identify side effects.

In Phase II trials, the experimental study drug or treatment is given to a larger group of people (100-300) to see if it is effective and to further evaluate its safety.

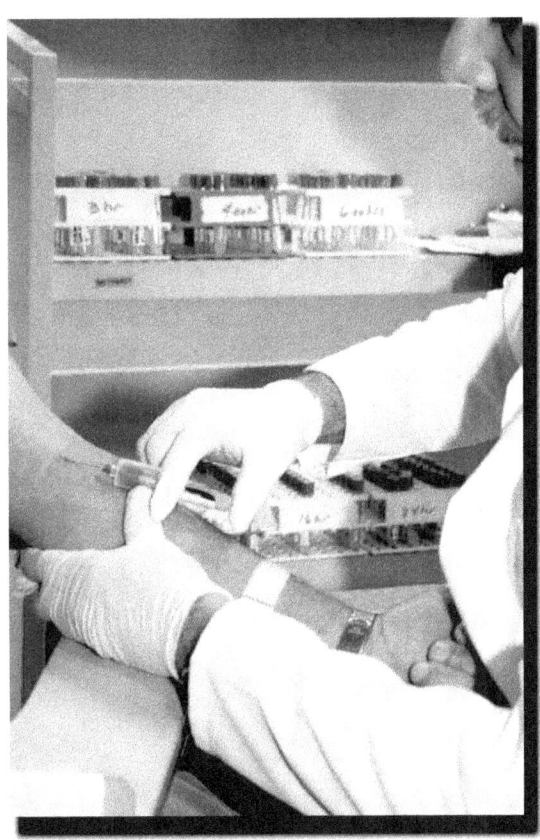

In Phase III trials, the experimental study drug or treatment is given to large groups of people (1,000-3,000) to confirm its effectiveness, monitor side effects, compare it to commonly used treatments, and collect information that will allow the experimental drug or treatment to be used safely.

In Phase IV trials, post marketing studies delineate additional information including the drug's risks, benefits, and optimal use.

What happens during a clinical trial?

The clinical trial process depends on the kind of trial being conducted. The clinical trial team includes doctors and nurses as well as social workers and other health care professionals. They check the health of the participant at the beginning of the trial, give specific instructions for participating in the trial, monitor the participant carefully during the trial, and stay in touch after the trial is completed.

Some clinical trials involve more tests and doctor visits than the participant would normally have for an illness or condition. For all types of trials, the participant works with a research team. Clinical trial participation is most successful when the protocol is carefully followed and there is frequent contact with the research staff.

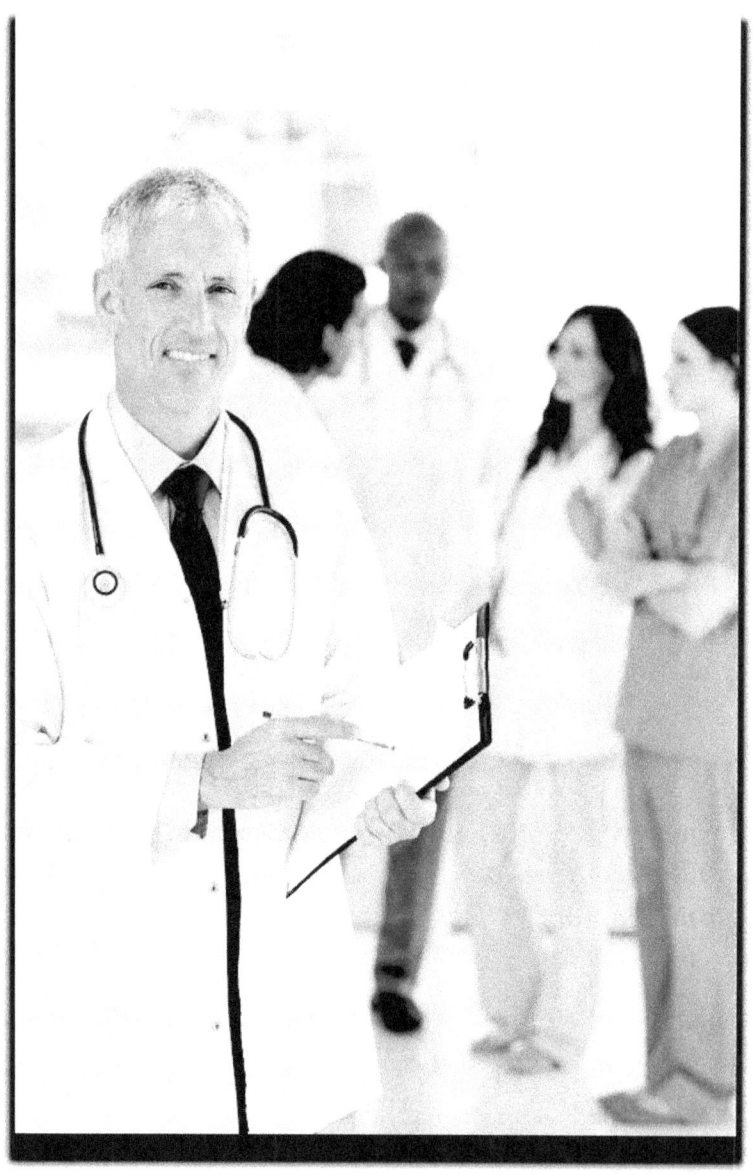

What is a clinical trial?

Although there are many definitions of clinical trials, they are generally considered to be biomedical or health-related research studies in human beings that follow a pre-defined protocol. ClinicalTrials.gov includes both interventional and observational types of studies. Interventional studies are those in which the research subjects are assigned by the investigator to a treatment or other intervention, and their outcomes are measured. Observational studies are those in which individuals are observed and their outcomes are measured by the investigators.

What is a control or control group?

A control is the standard by which experimental observations are evaluated. In many clinical trials, one group of patients will be given an experimental drug or treatment, while the control group is given either a standard treatment for the illness or a placebo.

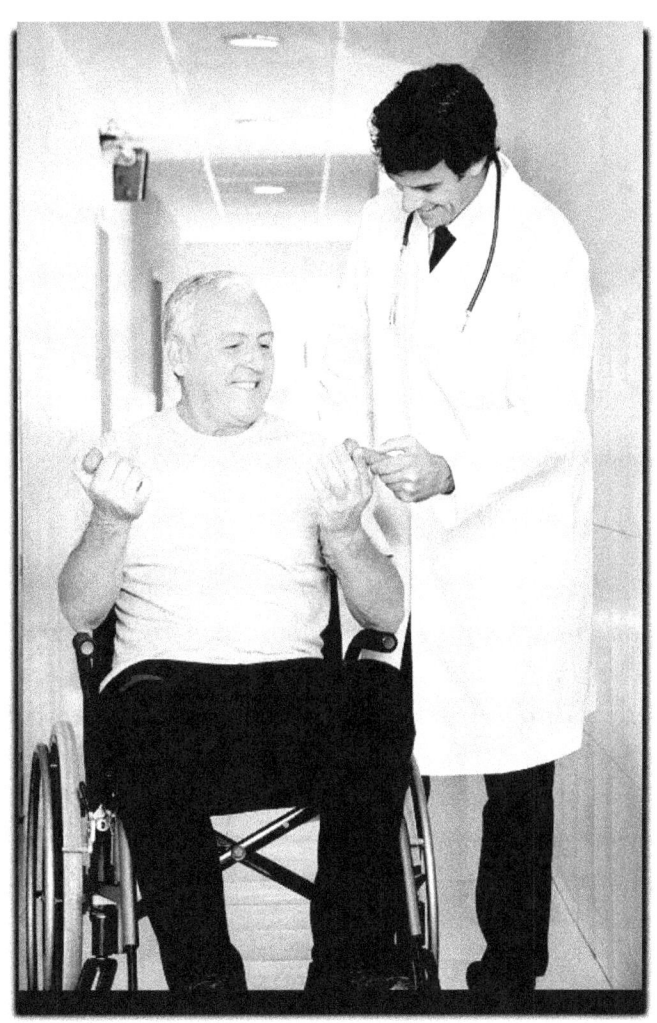

What is a placebo?

A placebo is an inactive pill, liquid, or powder that has no treatment value. In clinical trials, experimental treatments are often compared with placebos to assess the experimental treatment's effectiveness. In some studies, the participants in the control group will receive a placebo instead of an active drug or experimental treatment.

What is a protocol?

A protocol is a study plan on which all clinical trials are based. The plan is carefully designed to safeguard the health of the participants as well as answer specific research questions. A protocol describes what types of people may participate in the trial; the schedule of tests, procedures, medications, and dosages; and the length of the study. While in a clinical trial, participants following a protocol are seen regularly by the research staff to monitor their health and to determine the safety and effectiveness of their treatment.

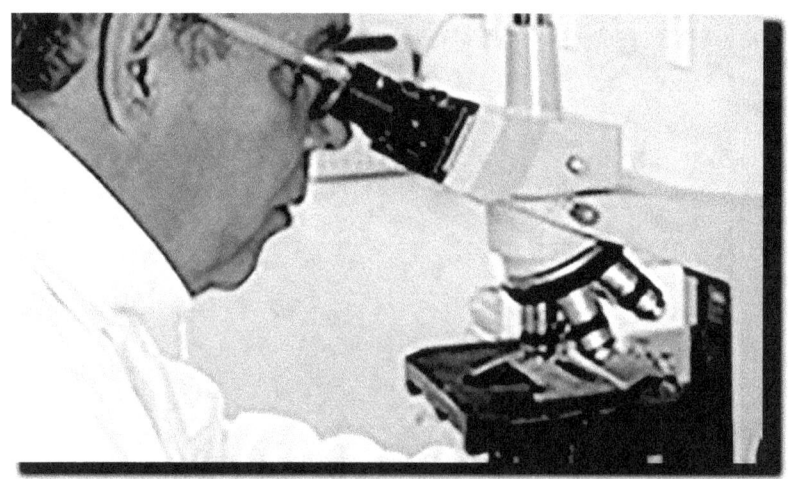

What is informed consent?

Informed consent is the process of learning the key facts about a clinical trial before deciding whether or not to participate. It is also a continuing process throughout the study to provide information for participants. To help someone decide whether or not to participate, the doctors and nurses involved in the trial explain the details of the study. If the participant's native language is not English, translation assistance can be provided. Then the research team provides an informed consent document that includes details about the study, such as its purpose, duration, required procedures, and key contacts. Risks and potential benefits are explained in the informed consent document. The participant then decides whether or not to sign the document. Informed consent is not a contract, and the participant may withdraw from the trial at any time.

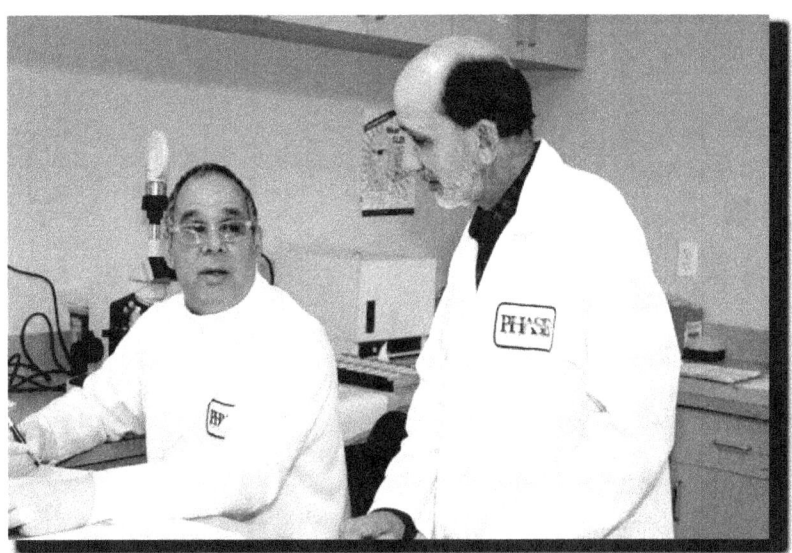

What is "expanded access"?

Expanded access is a means by which manufacturers make investigation new drugs available, under certain circumstances, to treat a patient(s) with a serious disease or condition who cannot participate in a controlled clinical trial.

Most human use of investigation new drugs takes place in controlled clinical trials conducted to assess the safety and efficacy of new drugs. Data from these trials are used to determine whether a drug is safe and effective, and serve as the basis for the drug marketing application. Sometimes, patients do not qualify for these controlled trials because of other health problems, age, or other factors, or are otherwise unable to enroll in such trials (e.g., a patient may not live sufficiently close to a clinical trial site).

For patients who cannot participate in a clinical trial of an investigation drug, but have a serious disease or condition that may benefit from treatment with the drug, FDA regulations enable manufacturers of such drugs to provide those patients access to the drug under certain situations, known as "expanded access." For example, the drug cannot expose patients to unreasonable risks given the severity of the disease to be treated and the patient does not have any other satisfactory therapeutic options (e.g., an approved drug that could be used to treat the patient's disease or condition). The manufacturer must be willing to make the drug available for expanded access use. The primary intent of expanded access is to provide treatment for a patient's disease or condition, rather than to collect data about the study drug.

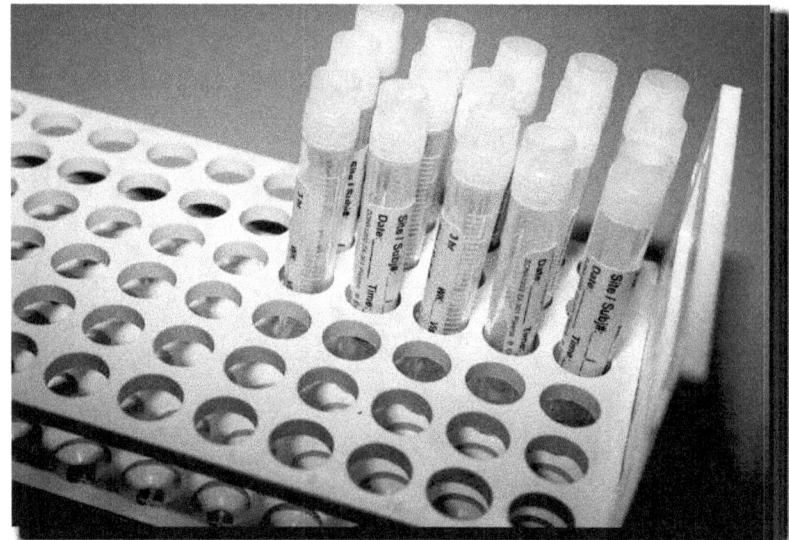

Some investigational drugs are available for treatment use from pharmaceutical manufacturers through expanded access programs listed in ClinicalTrials.gov. If you or a loved one is interested in treatment with an investigational drug under an expanded access protocol listed in ClinicalTrials.gov, review the protocol eligibility criteria and inquire at the Contact Information number. If there is not an expanded access protocol listed in ClinicalTrials.gov, you or your health care provider may contact a manufacturer of an investigational drug directly to ask about expanded access programs.

For additional information on expanded access programs, please see the FDA website at Access to Investigational Drugs.

What kind of preparation should a potential participant make for the meeting with the research coordinator or doctor?

Plan ahead and write down possible questions to ask.

Ask a friend or relative to come along for support and to hear the responses to the questions.

Every clinical trial in the U.S. must be approved and monitored by an Institutional Review Board (IRB) to make sure the risks are as low as possible and are worth any potential benefits. An IRB is an independent committee of physicians, statisticians, community advocates, and others that ensures that a clinical trial is ethical and the rights of study participants are protected. All institutions that conduct or support biomedical research involving people must, by federal regulation, have an IRB that initially approves and periodically reviews the research.

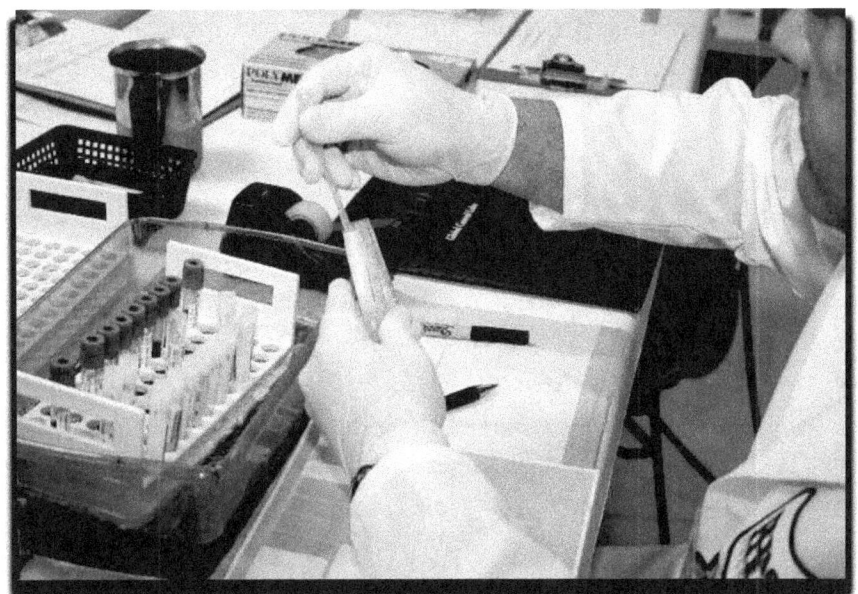

What should people consider before participating in a trial?

People should know as much as possible about the clinical trial and feel comfortable asking the members of the health care team questions about it, the care expected while in a trial, and the cost of the trial. The following questions might be helpful for the participant to discuss with the health care team. Some of the answers to these questions are found in the informed consent document.

Ideas for clinical trials usually come from researchers. After researchers test new therapies or procedures in the laboratory and in animal studies, the experimental treatments with the most promising laboratory results are moved into clinical trials. During a trial, more and more information is gained about an experimental treatment, its risks and how well it may or may not work.

Who can participate in a clinical trial?

All clinical trials have guidelines about who can participate.

Using inclusion/exclusion criteria is an important principle of medical research that helps to produce reliable results. The factors that allow someone to participate in a clinical trial are called "inclusion criteria" and those that disallow someone from participating are called "exclusion criteria". These criteria are based on such factors as age, gender, the type and stage of a disease, previous treatment history, and other medical conditions. Before joining a clinical trial, a participant must qualify for the study. Some research studies seek participants with illnesses or conditions to be studied in the clinical trial, while others need healthy participants. It is important to note that inclusion and exclusion criteria are not used to reject people personally.

Instead, the criteria are used to identify appropriate participants and keep them safe. The criteria help ensure that researchers will be able to answer the questions they plan to study.

Who sponsors clinical trials?

Clinical trials are sponsored or funded by a variety of organizations or individuals such as physicians, medical institutions, foundations, voluntary groups, and pharmaceutical companies, in addition to federal agencies such as the National Institutes of Health (NIH), the Department of Defense (DOD), and the Department of Veteran's Affairs (VA). Trials can take place in a variety of locations, such as hospitals, universities, doctors' offices, or community clinics.

Why participate in a clinical trial?

Participants in clinical trials can play a more active role in their own health care, gain access to new research treatments before they are widely available, and help others by contributing to medical research.

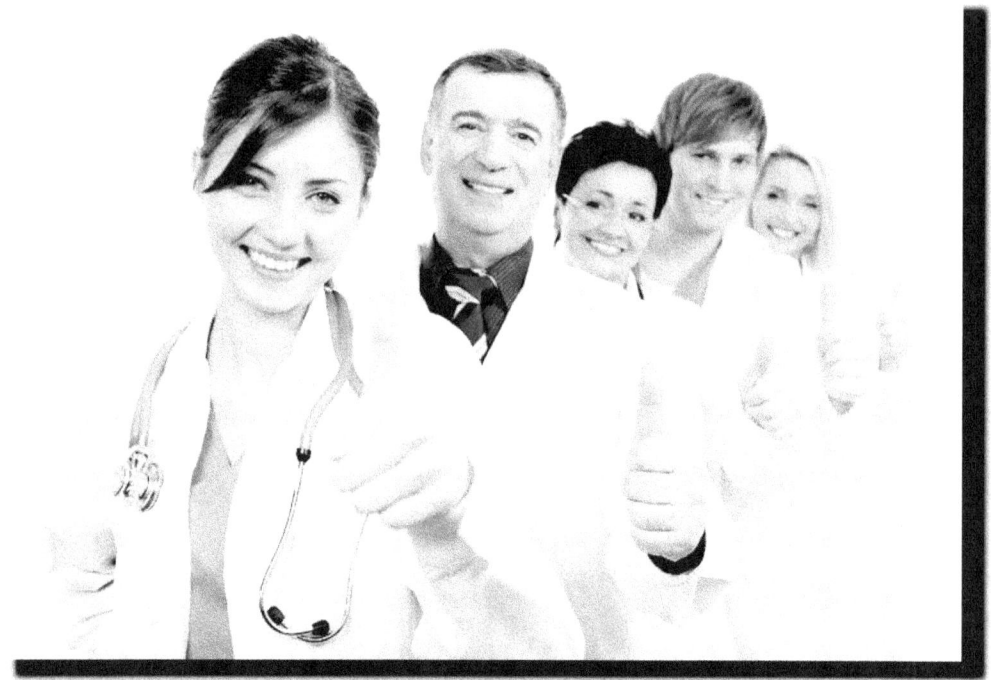

CRI Phase 1

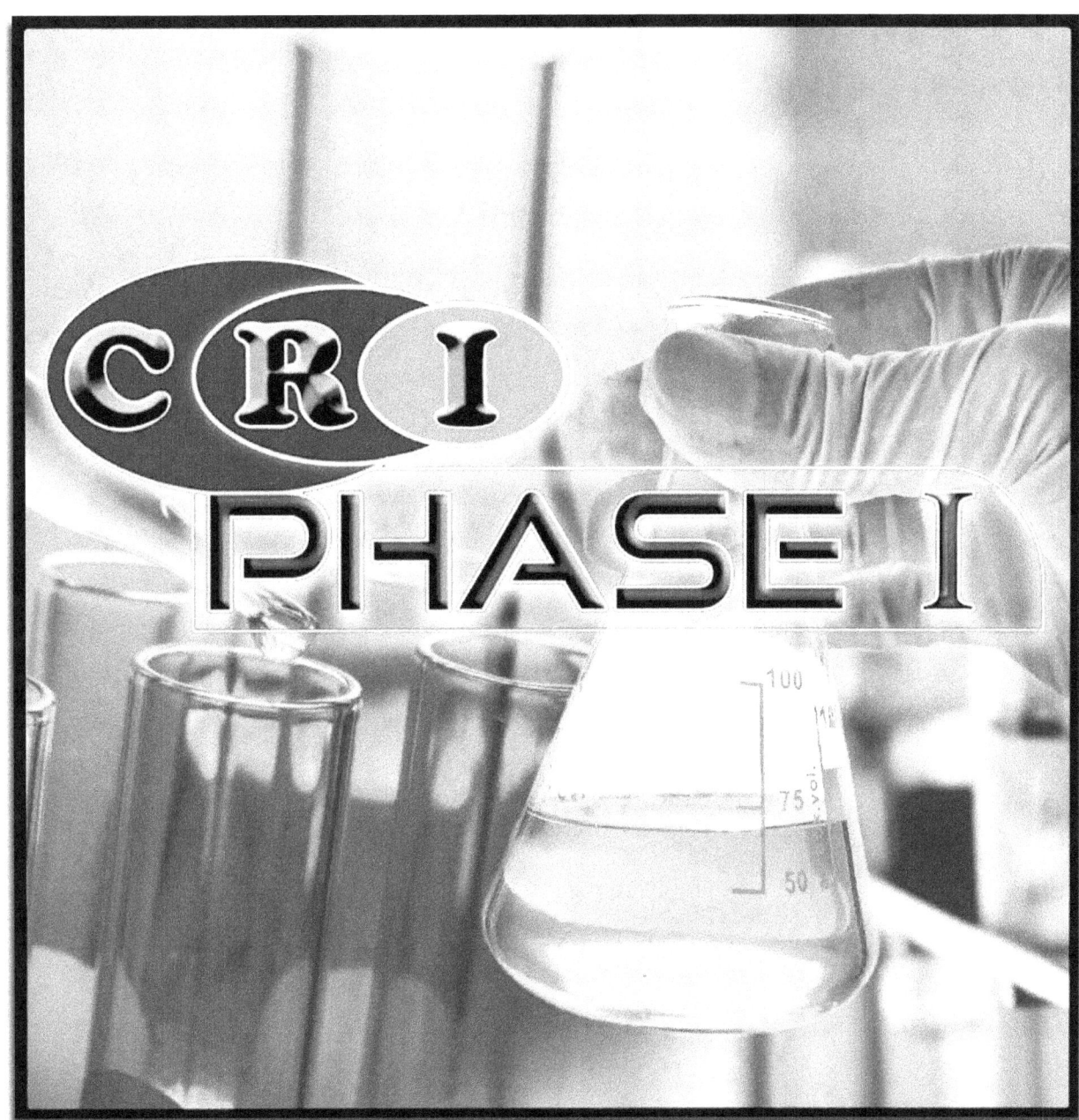

South East MD Clinical Skills Adviser
SEMDCSA
Dr. Hugo Romeu M.D.

SOUTH EAST MD CLINICAL
SKILL ADVISER
SEMDCSA

dr.hugoromeu@yahoo.com

SEMDCSA

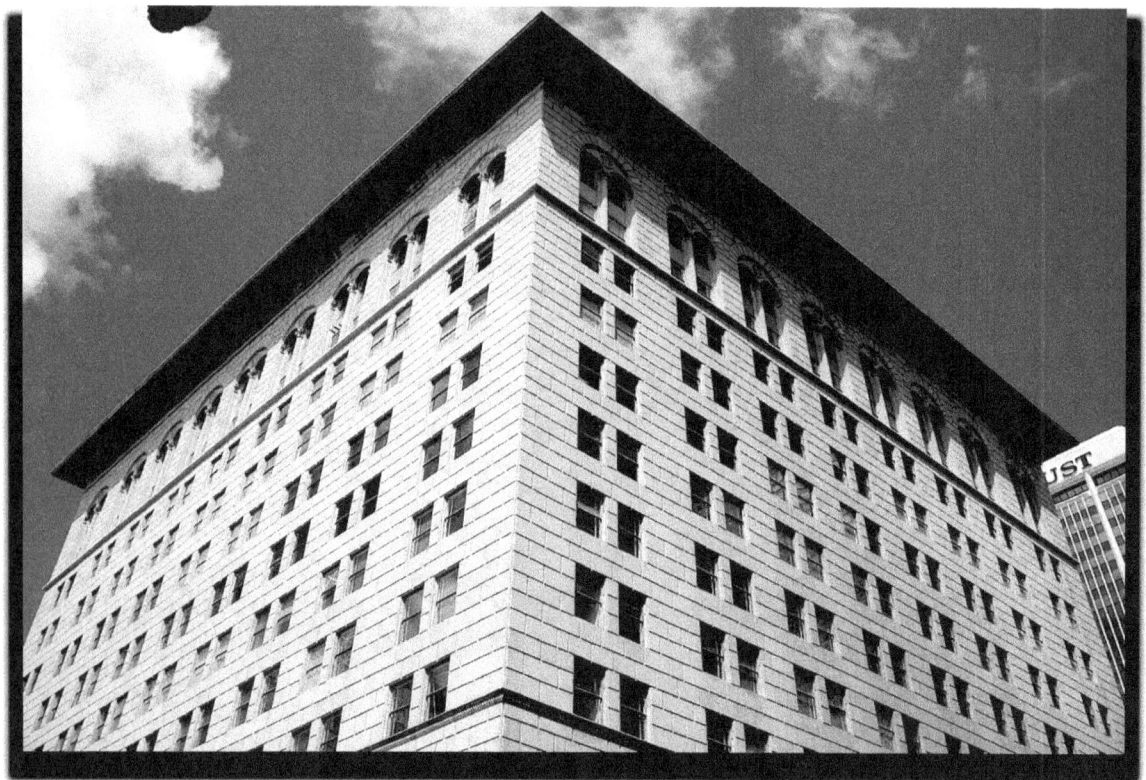

25 Southeast Second Avenue Suite 818
Miami, Fl 33131
Office (305) 642 7011
Cell (305) 281 3633

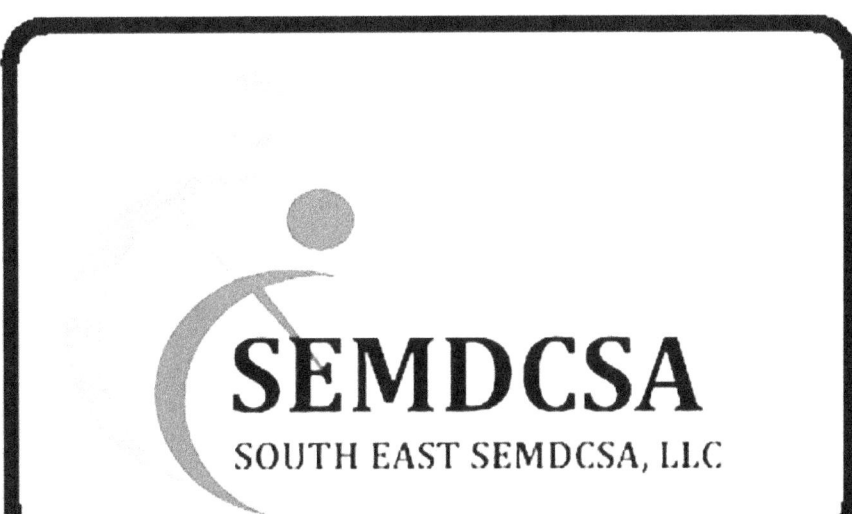

South East MD Clinical Advisors

International MD Clinical Skills Advisors Our program is tailored specifically for the International Medical Student or Physician. This program is a joint effort between a wide array of Medical Schools, Hospitals, and Training Facilities which are all dedicated and certified by Accrediting Bodies in the U.S.A. We have different programs based on the individual desire of our client, the student or physician. The first step is to clarify the exact intended desire. For example; Is it clinical exposure to a U.S. Hospital and routine practice of medicine? Is it to polish your skills and return to your country? Do you wish to obtain credit for a clinical rotation, or are you looking for a certificate of completion and recommendation? We need to know what the exit objective is for each individual. Whatever the reason for applying to our program, we guarantee a maximum quality exposure to the best facilities and professional expertise in training physicians. Upon leaving our program the aspirant will testify to other potential clients the well rounded and satisfying outcome of the MD Clinical Skills Advisor rotation. The length is optional. We have one month basic exposure programs, and can provide a 48 week rotation which includes accredited rotations in Internal

Medicine, Family Practice, Surgery, Ob/Gyn, Pediatrics and Psychiatry. Also available is USMLE step 1 and 2 preparation. Upon the successful completion each candidate will receive a certificate of completion and 2 letters of recommendation. Our success is predicated by the attendees future accomplishments, and our track record is well proven. For further information contact: SEMDCSA International Affairs Phone/ fax email

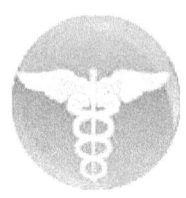

SEMDCSA is the offspring of two physicians dedicated to Graduate level Education

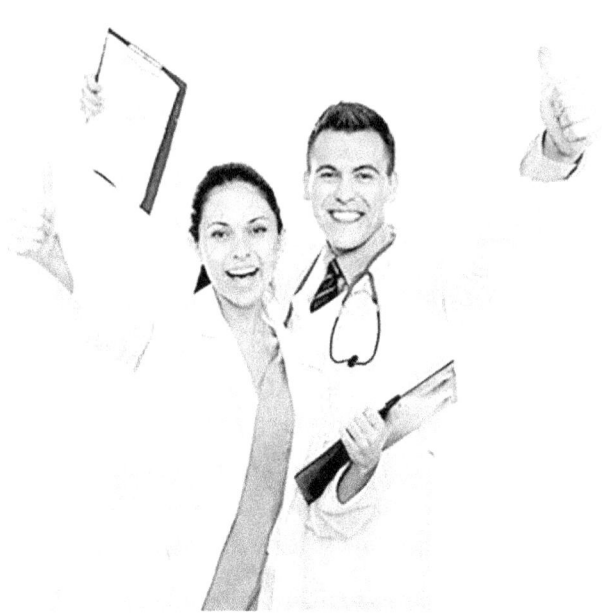

SEMDCSA is the offspring of two physicians dedicated to Graduate level Education for over a combined 20 years. Together Dr. Hugo Romeu and Dr. Don Dolce have been involved in Medical Student Training for prestigious institutions on every continent. Together they have their hands in the development of over 2000 medical students of which nearly 80 % are currently practicing medicine in the U.S.A.

SEMDCSA is currently focused in South Florida

SEMDCSA is currently focused in South Florida, where there are numerous Medical Schools and Teaching Hospitals. Another rich source for hands on exposure to the real world of medical practice is the utilization of public health care facilities laden with Post Graduate Residents in Specialty Training, and scores of Medical Students from both the U.S.A. and abroad.

Although each maintains their individual educational projects

Although each maintains their individual educational projects, SEMDCSA is a humble attempt to culminate the fruits of their prior experience, into a powerhouse high level teaching institution. The two most important factors in guaranteeing a suitable infrastructure for success, and this is gaged by student development into licensed physicians, is contracting with Accredited Facilities and Dedicated Physicians.

The first step is an application

The Attendant Physicians which take care of each student are hand-picked to match the objective desire of each individual applicant. Our staff is ready to assist each student with housing, transportation and guidance. The first step is an application and telephone interview to assess which program suits the aspiring physician. Please fill out the following application at info@305MD.com

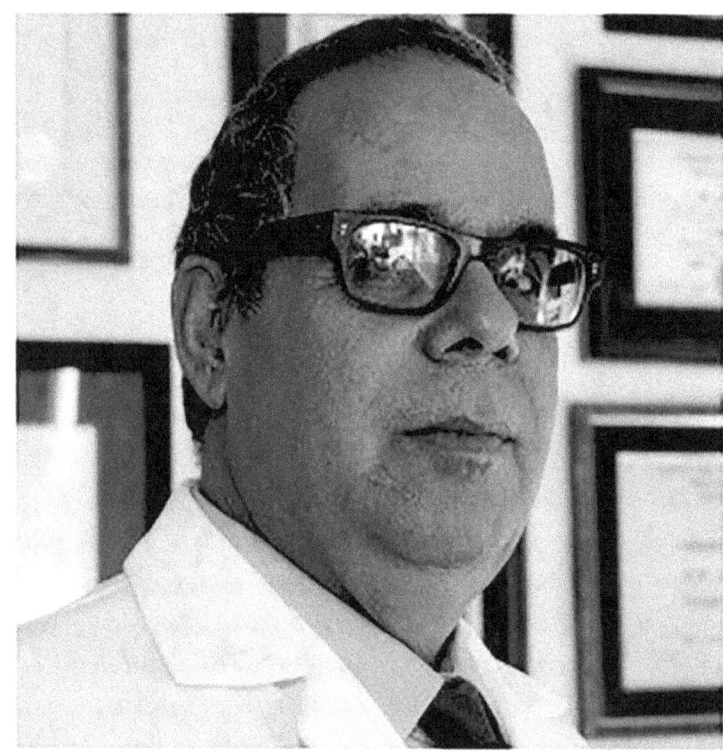

Dr. Hugo Romeu, MD
Pathologist

Medical Core Rotation Requirements

SEMDCSA is currently partnering with a wide array of International and National Institutions to provide both accredited and preparatory courses for Medical Students and Graduates seeking a Post Graduate position. Our requirements for an interview and placement are: To: 3rd or 4th year Medical Students • Completed application form • Letter of good standing from your medical school. • Immunization records • Recommendation letter (2) • Copy of passport (Information page only) • 2 (2X2) passport size photo • $300.00 Application fee, Payable to: Romeu Clinical Enterprises • Tuition: will be calculated based on requested number of weeks ; the range is from $500.00 to $700.00 per week.

- *Completed application form*
- *Copy of Medical Doctorate Degree*
- *Copy of USMLE Scores (If applicable)*
- *Malpractice insurance*
- *Immunization records*
- *Recommendation letter (2)*
- *Copy of passports (Information page only)*
- *2 (2X2) passport size photo*
- *$400.00 Application fee, Payable to: _____*
- *Tuition: will be calculated based on requested number of weeks ; varies from $500.00 to $700.00*

US Requirements

Your attending will guide you through the culture of U.S. healthcare, helping you navigate the black-and-white rules as well as subtleties that every U.S. medical graduate learns during medical school.

During each clinical experience, you will learn and hone skills in documenting methods such as charting, SOAP notes, admitting and discharge orders, and electronic as well as handwritten data systems.

You'll be encouraged to conduct oral case presentations and share physical findings, and communicate with patients and their families, your colleagues, and the medical staff.

While covered by extensive medical liability insurance, you will obtain the experience needed to become an asset to any U.S. residency program.

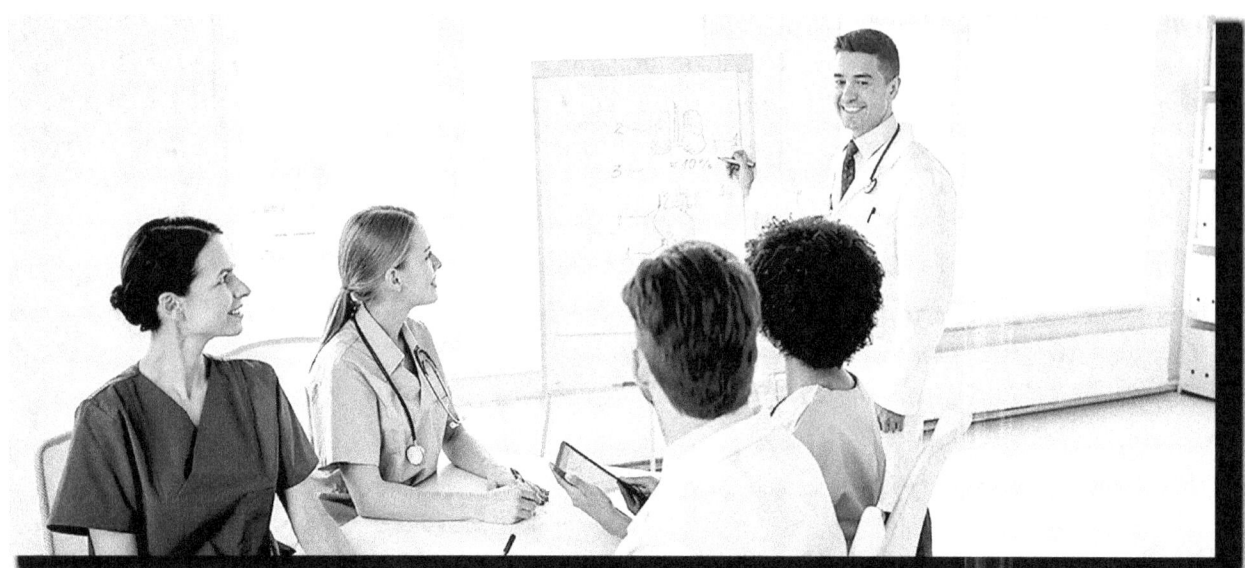

In any regard, we know everyone likes to talk to the "right person our departments is highly trained and specialized, so although we are always happy to help" the first time around. Our teams are:

- *Enrollment: For initial clinical schedules and new or additional clinical blocks or services*

- *Career Development: For enrollment processing, document collection, document revision, career counseling, and medical branding*

- *Medical Development: For specific questions regarding clinical blocks, clinical site requirements, and changes in your schedule*

Your attending will guide you through the culture of U.S. healthcare, helping you navigate the black-and-white rules as well as subtleties that every U.S. medical graduate learns during medical school.

The Ob-Gyn curriculum provides exposure to many aspects of primary care. Within in allocated time frame students will see only a portion of the many diseases, disorders, and procedures that obstetricians and gynecologists manage. consequently, students are responsible for independent preparation for standardized Shelf and board examinations.

As in every medical rotation, the trainee must become the consummate professional Demonstrating respect, compassion, integrity, and altruism in relationships with patients, families, and colleagues.
All medical professionals must be empathetic, demonstrating sensitivity and responsiveness to the gender, age, culture, religion, sexual preference, socioeconomic status, beliefs, behaviors, and disabilities of patients and colleagues.

Students are required to complete one case based presentation, including an in depth Discussion of one or more aspects of the case (e.g. a presenting symptom or sign, a diagnostic category or management issue) that you want to learn more about during your rotation.

The actual case chosen should be based on a patient the student personally evaluated in either the inpatient or outpatient setting.

The presentation will be given to the Ob-Gyn Attending Physician/Preceptor and any other members of the medical team (e.g. medical students, interns, residents).

The presentation should be about 15-20 minutes in length and should be accompanied by handouts including a written description of the case and an evidence based discussion of the topic to be presented with a list of the recent literature used to obtain information for the discussion.

The literature could include material from journal articles, national guidelines, professional publications and web sites such as the American College of Obstetricians and Gynecologists (ACOG) or recent textbook.

Generally speaking, all rotations listed above should be completed before electives are taken. In some instances, however, electives may be taken before all core rotations are completed, but only with the permission of the Dean of Clinical Studies and only if the related parent core rotation has already been completed successfully.

Rotation	Type	Weeks Required
Internal Medicine	Core	12
Surgery	Core	12
Ob/Gyn	Core	6
Pediatrics	Core	6
Psychiatry	Core	6
Family Medicine	Core	6
Emergency Medicine	Elective	2
Pediatrics	Elective	3 or 6
Internal Medicine	Elective	0 or 3
Infectious Disease	Elective	2
Radiology	Elective	2
Nuclear Medicine	Elective	1*
Pathology	Elective	1*
Dermatology	Elective	0 / 2**
Choice	Elective	4 / 6**
Rehab	Elective	1*
Oncology	Elective	1*
Dentistry	Elective	1*
ENT	Elective	2***
Neurology	Elective	2
Neurosurgery	Elective	2
Ophthalmology	Elective	2
Anesthesia / ICU	Elective	2
Orthopedic Surgery	Elective	1*
TOTAL REQUIRED	**82 weeks**	

Affiliation with Graduate and Post Graduate level

RRL takes pride in their affiliation with Graduate and Post Graduate level affiliations. We are anxious to assist our clinical partners with understanding the physiopathology and mechanics of Laboratory Medicine. Our Clinical companions are welcome to visit our facility, and we will prepare an in-service training sessions to fully understand your own clinical aspirations. We offer a 4 week course to all levels of professionals; from Board Certified Physicians, Ph.D. Candidates, Lab technologists and Clinical Coordinators. The objective is to get a firsthand experience into the esoteric world of clinical laboratory research. Our clerkship is designed to provide the clinical experiences and didactics to familiarize you with the core competencies of obstetrical and gynecologic care. Obstetrics and gynecology is a dynamic specialty that blends elements of surgery, medicine, and primary preventive care into a single practice. The primary goals of the clerkship are to better understand the work of primary care physicians, their interactions with community and other health professionals, common primary care conditions, and strategies for enhancing communication with patients.

INTERNATIONAL MEDICINE PROGRAMS

SUMMER RESEARCH & MEDICAL ENRICHMENT PROGRAM

PROGRAM OVERVIEW

SEMDCSA, South East M.D. Clinical Skills Advisors, will offer the opportunity for talented 3rd and 4th year international students in health sciences, graduated of Medicines School and specialist in the medical field, to participate in a summer research and medical training. Through this program, students and physicians will have access to medical and research enrichment opportunities with practical of recognizes doctors and several Hospitals in Miami and gain exposure to the US medical education, research, and healthcare system.

In addition, this program will provide students and professionals with workshops and activities that will enhance research skills and provide medical enrichment opportunities and professional development.

This provides a unique stepping for students motivated to pursue graduate medical education and training in the United States.

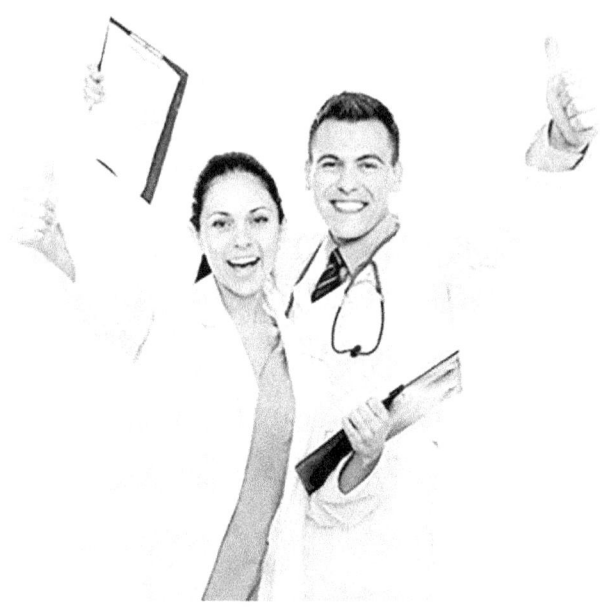

OBJECTIVES & OUTCOMES

Through this program, participants will have the opportunity to achieve the following learning objectives:

- *Gain exposure to resources and experts at an internationally recognized institution .*
- *Obtain hands-on research experience in state-of-the-art laboratories*
- *Gain skills in the research processes and presentation of research projects*
- *Develop strong cross-cultural skills and improve English language skills*
- *Gain first-hand knowledge of American medical education, research, and healthcare systems .*
- *Enhance the credentials of those students and/or professionals who are motivated to pursue graduate medical education and training in the United States.*
- *Participate through service, enrichment, and social events^*
- *Create a network of professional contacts for future support in educational and professional endeavors*
- *Letter of completion from Schools of Medicine and Health Sciences in South Florida .*

PROGRAM DESCRIPTION

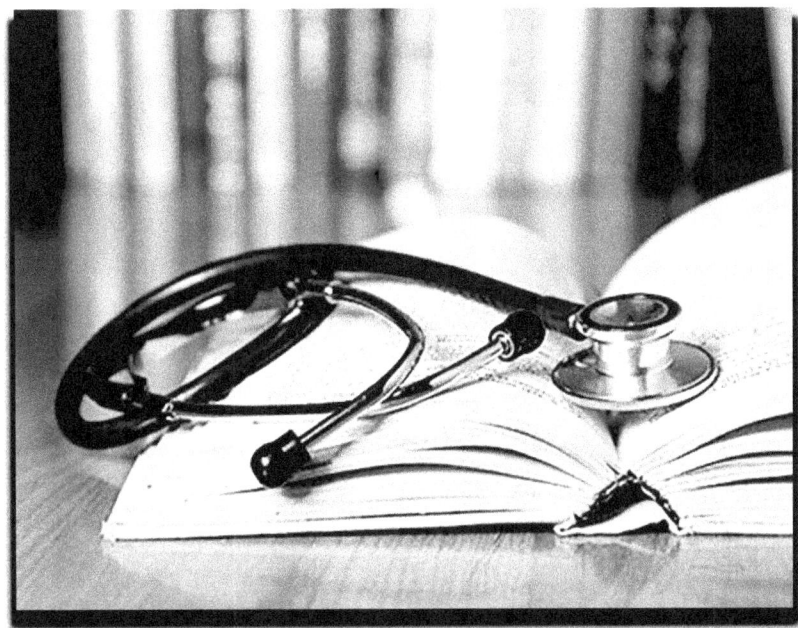

The curriculum includes the following components:

1. Mentorship in a Research Project: The student's primary focus will be working with a mentor who will include in their current research projects.
The faculty mentor will provide guidance on best practices for research, design, and methodology.

2. Research Skill Building: Students will attend workshops on research process, scientific manuscript writing, presentation skills, poster design, laboratory safety and other relevant topics.

3. Medical Enrichment: Students will be exposed to how basic sciences and clinical medicine are practiced at enrichment activities include microbiology, pathology, and radiology lab tours; epidemiology lectures; conversations with basic sciences and clinical faculty; patient experience and hospital environment; etc.

4. Professional Development and Cultural Enrichment Workshops: A variety of workshops will be imparted to meet the students or professionals development needs. These workshops include English writing, career guidance, working in groups, library resources, CV and personal statement writing, culture, stereotypes, and biases, professionalism, etc..

5. Evaluation: All students will be evaluated on their attendance, participation, and performance throughout the program. They will also be asked to provide feedback on the overall program and their experiences. Letters of Completion will be granted at the end of the summer to students or professionals who successfully complete the program.

6. Social Activities: Outside of the classroom, the group will be encouraged to explore and take advantage of the vibrancy and significance of our location and campus environment. Students can participate in cultural and recreational activities across campus and Washington, D.C. including the White House, Capitol, Smithsonian Museums, government agencies (e.g. Library of Congress, Supreme Court), historical monuments and international organization headquarters (e.g. World Bank), and sporting events (e.g. Washington Nationals Baseball).

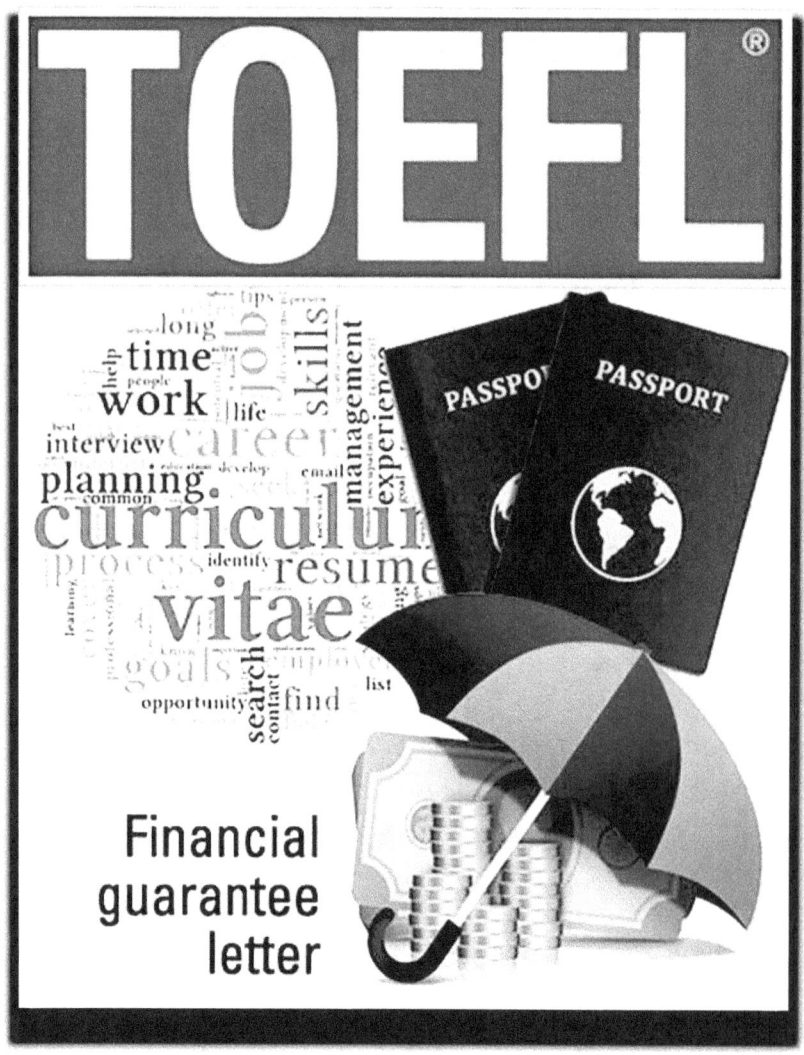

APPLICATION PROCESS AND SELECTION CRITERIA

Interested and qualified students must submit the following documents in one PDF packet to www.SEMDCSA.com OR www.305MD.com in order to be considered for admission:

- *Curriculum Vitae*

- *Copy of Passport*

- *English Proficiency (TOEFL >90 score report or Skype interview and writing samples)*

- *Dean's Letter of Good Standing*

- *One Letter of Recommendation (from a faculty member at the applicant's home school)*

- *Medical School Transcripts*

- *One-page objective statement (12-point Font Times New Roman, single-spaced detailing the applicant's future goals and objectives for research and clinical training)*

- *Financial guarantee or sponsorship letter (if applicable)*

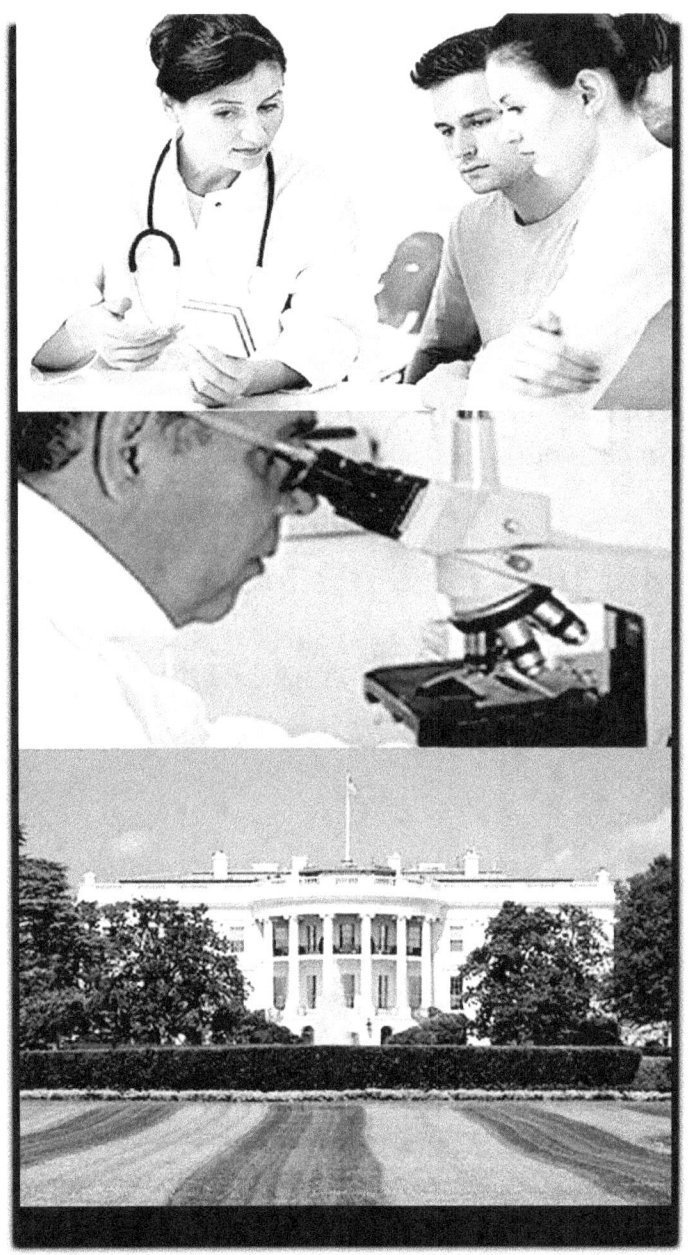

Acceptance is based on applicant's qualifications and availability. Applicants should apply as soon as possible as space is limited and visa processing times may vary.

Applicants must have completed their 3rd or 4th year (of a six-year program) or be graduated of medical school.

COST

The program cost for each student will be informed directly to the applicant. A non-refundable seat deposit of $500 will be due when the applicant is accepted into the program to confirm their participation. The deposit will apply to the total tuition of the program, and full payment will be due upon acceptance and receipt of invoice.

- *Students will be responsible for covering their own airfare, transportation, housing, health insurance, immunizations, and daily living expenses.*

- *Each student must obtain his or her own visa. Students are responsible for meeting all costs, deadlines, and other requirements associated with obtaining a visa.*

- *SEMDCSA will facilitate students who are seeking on housing. We will also provide guidance about travel to and living in Miami.*

Internal Medicine Rotation

Internal Medicine core curriculum provides exposure to many aspects of internal medicine. However in a limited time frame students will see only a portion of the many diseases, disorders, and procedures that Internal Medicine physicians manage.

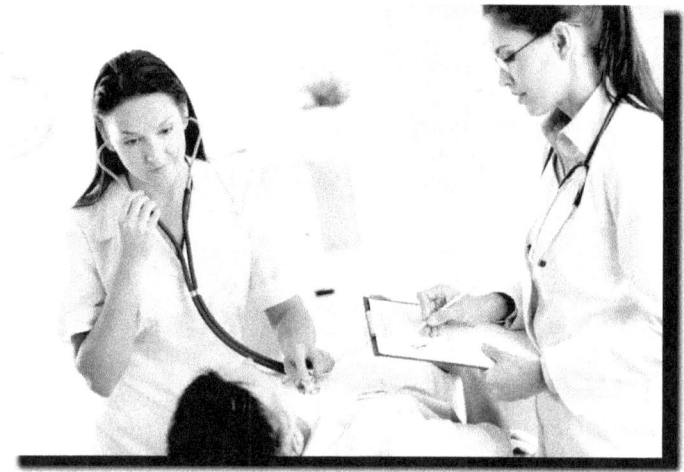

Consequently, student are responsible for independent preparation for standardized Shelf and Board examinations.

-Each student is responsible for going into this essential rotation with the fundamental knowledge required to maximize the experience.

We recommend that each of the following topics be sought out during the clinical rotation:

- *Acute Coronary Syndrome*
- *Acute Renal Failure*
- *Alcohol and Drug Withdrawal*
- *Asthma*
- *Cardiac Arrhythmias*
- *Cellulitis*
- *COPD*
- *Community Acquired Pneumonia*
- *CHF*
- *Delirium and Dementia*
- *DM*
- *GI Bleed*
- *Hospital Acquired Pneumonia*
- *Pain Management*
- *PE, DVT*
- *Perioperative Medicine*
- *Sepsis Syndrome*
- *Stroke*
- *UTI*
- *VTE*
- *Skin & Soft Tissue Infections*
- *Abdominal bleeding and pain*
- *Altered mental status*
- *Anemia*
- *Diabetes Mellitus*
- *Hypertension*
- *Infectious Diseases*
- *Community Acquired Pneumonia*
- *Sepsis*
- *Kidney Failure; acute and chronic*
- *Liver failure*
- *Low Back Pain*

Keep in mind that Internal Medicine is in fact the in depth intellectual understanding of the mechanism of disease, and the practical diagnostic regimen to achieve the optimum therapeutic remedy.

Gynecology & Obstetrics Rotation

The Ob-Gyn curriculum provides exposure to many aspects of primary care. Within in allocated time frame students will see only a portion of the many diseases, disorders, and procedures that obstetricians and gynecologists manage. consequently, students are responsible for independent preparation for standardized Shelf and board examinations. As in every medical rotation, the trainee must become the consummate professional demonstrating respect, compassion, integrity, and altruism in relationships with patients, families, and colleagues. All medical professionals must be empathetic, demonstrating sensitivity and responsiveness to the gender, age, culture, religion, sexual preference, socioeconomic status, beliefs, behaviors, and disabilities of patients and colleagues. Students are required to complete one case based presentation, including an in depth discussion of one or more aspects of the case (e.g. a presenting symptom or sign, a diagnostic category or management issue) that you want to learn more about during your rotation.

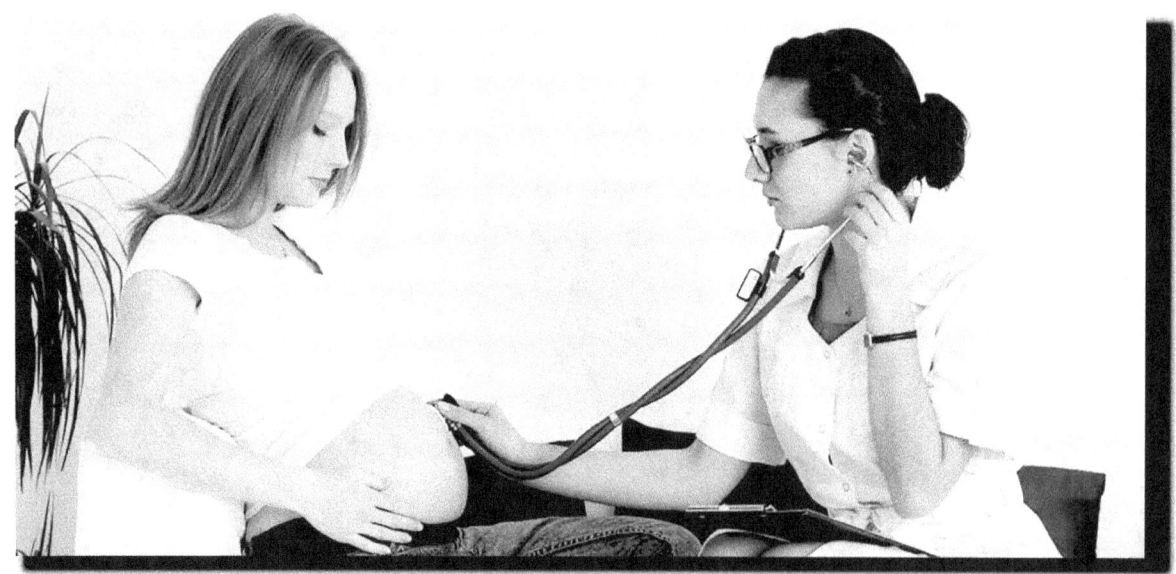

The actual case chosen should be based on a patient the student personally evaluated in either the inpatient or outpatient setting.

The presentation will be given to the Ob-Gyn Attending Physician/Preceptor and any other members of the medical team (e.g. medical students, interns, residents).

The presentation should be about 15-20 minutes in length and should be accompanied by handouts including a written description of the case and an evidence based discussion of the topic to be presented with a list of the recent literature used to obtain information for the discussion.

The literature could include material from journal articles, national guidelines, professional publications and web sites such as the American College of Obstetricians and Gynecologists (ACOG) or recent textbook

Our clerkship is designed to provide the clinical experiences and didactics to familiarize you with the core competencies of obstetrical and gynecologic care. Obstetrics and gynecology is a dynamic specialty that blends elements of surgery, medicine, and primary preventive care into a single practice.

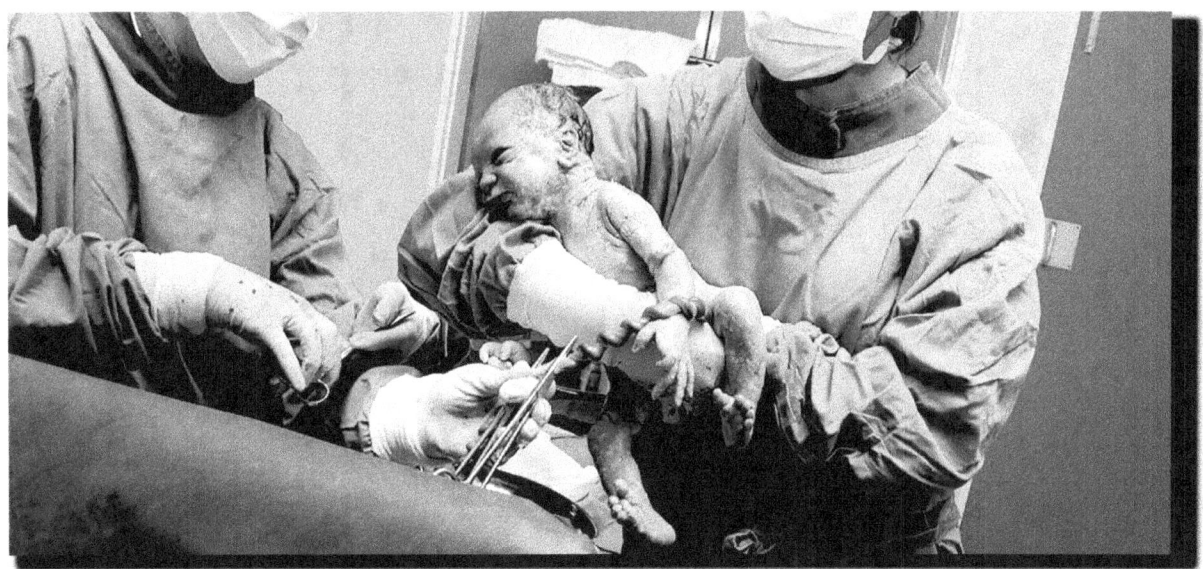

The primary goals of the clerkship are to better understand the work of primary care physicians, their interactions with community and other health professionals, common primary care conditions, and strategies for enhancing communication with patients.
Your attending will guide you through the culture of U.S. healthcare, helping you navigate the black-and-white rules as well as subtleties that every U.S. medical graduate learns during medical school.

During each clinical experience, you will learn and hone skills in documenting methods such as charting, SOAP notes, admitting and discharge orders, and electronic as well as handwritten data systems. You'll be encouraged to conduct oral case presentations and share physical findings, and communicate with patients and their families, your colleagues, and the medical staff. While covered by extensive medical liability insurance, you will obtain the experience needed to become an asset to any U.S. residency program.

in any regard, we know everyone likes to talk to the "right person our departments is highly trained and specialized, so although we are always happy to help" the first time around.

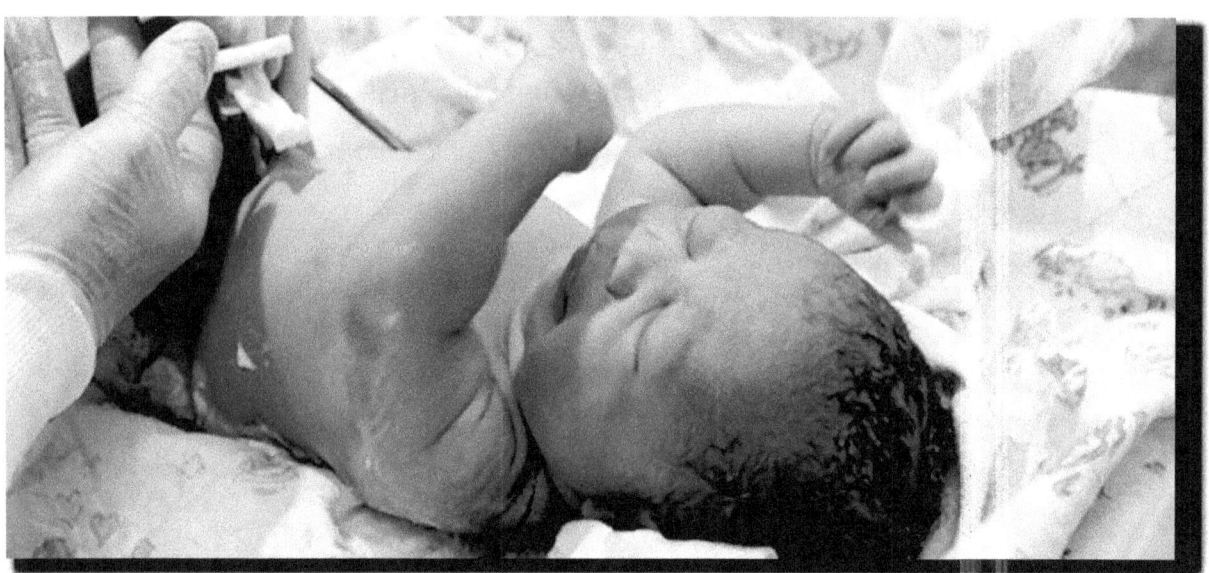

Our teams are:

- *Enrollment: For initial clinical schedules and new or additional clinical blocks or services*
- *Career Development: For enrollment processing, document collection, document revision, career counseling, and medical branding*
- *Medical Development: For specific questions regarding clinical blocks, clinical site requirements, and changes in your schedule*

Your attending will guide you through the culture of U.S. healthcare, helping you navigate the black-and-white rules as well as subtleties that every U.S. medical graduate learns during medical school.

Generally speaking, all rotations listed above should be completed before electives are taken. In some instances, however, electives may be taken before all core rotations are completed, but only with the permission of the Dean of Clinical Studies and only if the related parent core rotation has already been completed successfully.

Psichiatry Core Rotation

Our goals are to provide an overview of psychiatry, under the guidance of a Board Certified Psychiatrist. The trainee must learn how to recognize and manage psychiatric problems. In addition we hope to enhance your understanding of patient physician relationship. Whatever specialty a physician chooses, a basic understanding of psychiatry goes a long way to making the trainee a better doctor.

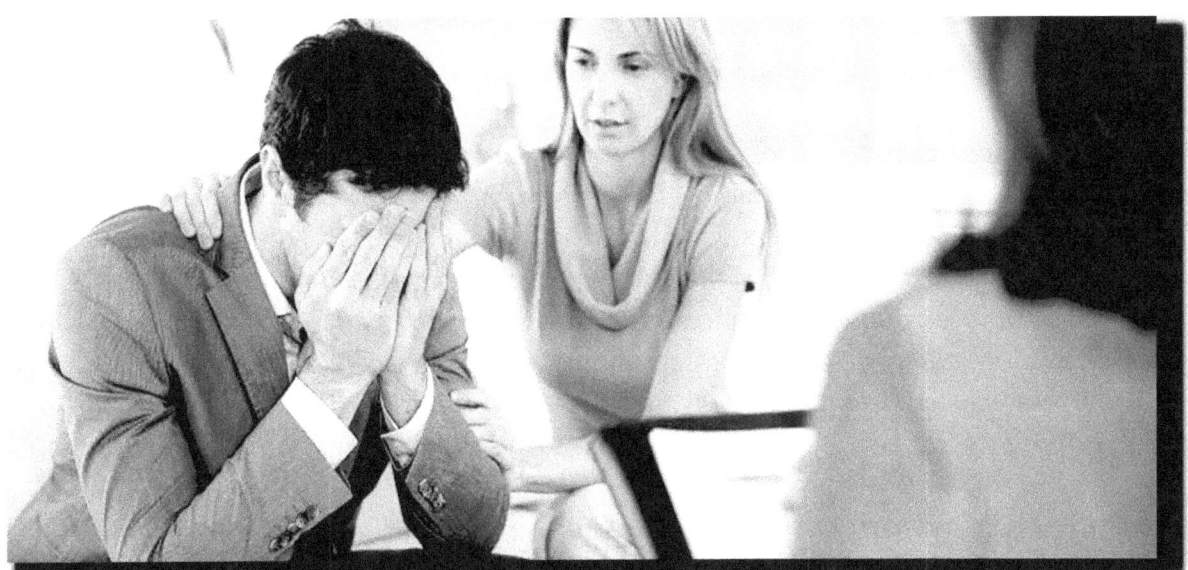

CLINICAL ACTIVITIES :

You will be assigned an attending for each rotation and will be working with residents on the same unit. The attending and resident physicians will orient you to their services, each of which has its own schedule for rounds, teaching conferences, team meetings, and therapy sessions. Services vary in the responsibility assigned to students. Be sure you understand what your role is to be, and what expectations your attending and resident physicians have for you.

PATIENT LOG

*The patient logbook is an opportunity for you to receive immediate feedback on your patient evaluations and allows you to gain knowledge and skills in the field of Psychiatry. You should complete a minimum of **6** out of **9** patient problems listed. The logbook is worth 25% of your final grade including the final H&P write up, so students should apply themselves in this area. Make copies of these pages and get as many done as possible before they are due so as to be able to turn the best ones in.*

Adult Core Rotations

Adult Inpatient

The Adult Services program provides inpatient mental health services to those with severe and chronic mental illnesses, The program adheres to a bio-psycho-social approach to mental illness . About half of the patients are diagnosed with schizophrenia, about a quarter are diagnosed with mood disorders, and the rest hold a variety of diagnoses such as personality, eating, and anxiety disorders. Patients with such difficulties as deafness, substance abuse, and medical complications are also treated on this service. Along with chronic and severe physical health issues and all such challenges are a part of the treatment mission and assignment.

Adult patients are typically drawn from urban setting and many of them come from stressed socio-economic living arrangements and some are experiencing homelessness. A good number of patients are forensic patients as well, both in the categories of outdate from correctional facilities or as needing to be restored to competency for legal procedures.

The intern will join a multidisciplinary treatment team on one of these units and assume a wide range of clinical activities focusing on participation in specialized patient education programs for those diagnosed with such chronic disorders as schizophrenia, mood disorders, or borderline personality disorder. The intern may also have the opportunity to supervise psychology graduate students and to initiate and/or collaborate with ongoing research projects. Research results have focused on the treatment of those who are deaf, those with Borderline Personality Disorder, and treatment outcomes.

Several supervisors are available to be assigned as intern supervision. The Director of Training will make the assignment of the intern's unit and supervisor based on intern interests among a range of factors, so a wide variety of experience is available for trainees.

The psychology intern will work with the supervisory psychologist in the assessment of newly admitted patients, provide consultation to the treatment team regarding behavioral management, and function in the role of primary therapist for select patients. In the role of primary therapist, a psychology intern typically provides individual therapy and coordinates the efforts of other members of a multidisciplinary treatment team. The intern may also participate in and co-lead therapy groups and unit meetings. Psychology interns will be exposed to pharmacotherapy issues and assist the psychiatrists and the treatment team in the process of evaluating and potentially reducing the medical regimen of patients.

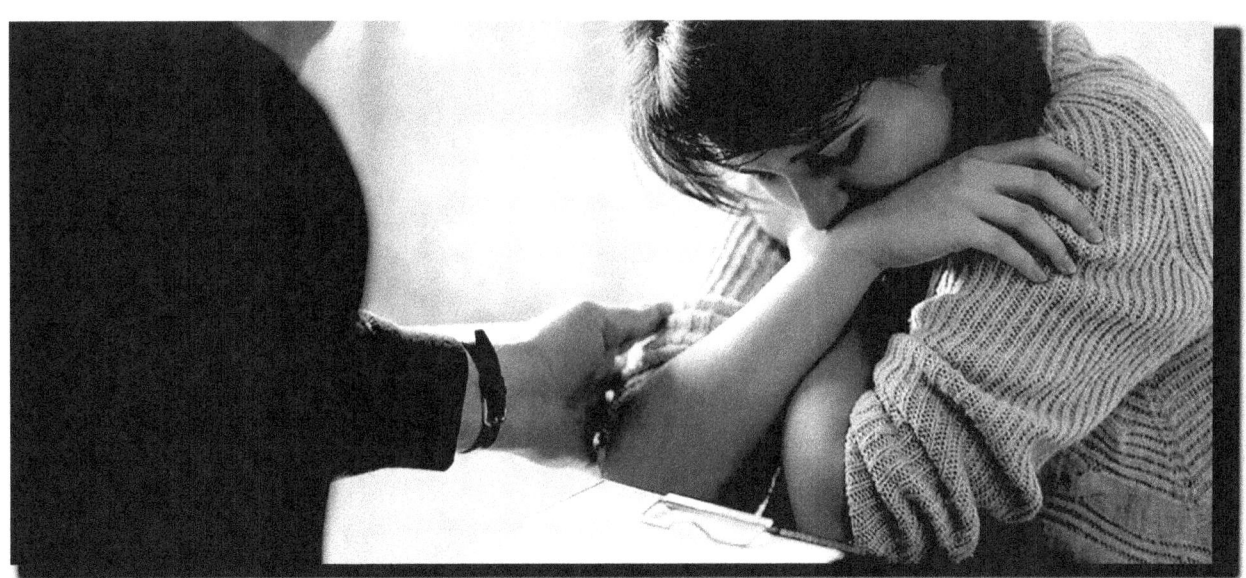

Adult Outpatient

The adult outpatient rotation takes place at the Adult Psychiatry Clinic and Study Centerr is a tertiary care facility with nationally and internationally recognized programs in specialized medical care.

General psychiatry residents as well as psychology interns rotate through the clinic, The clinic offers psychiatric services, including consultation-liaison services, and outpatient psychological testing and treatment.

The clinic is staffed by IU faculty physicians and psychologists, social workers, and trainees in each of these disciplines. Clinicians specialize in the treatment of mood disorders, anxiety disorders, personality disorders, geriatric disorders, behavioral health issues, and women's issues.

Interns on this rotation may have the opportunity to conduct clinical interviews and diagnostic assessments, provide individual and group psychotherapy, receive individual and group supervision, and provide supervised supervision to doctoral students in clinical psychology.

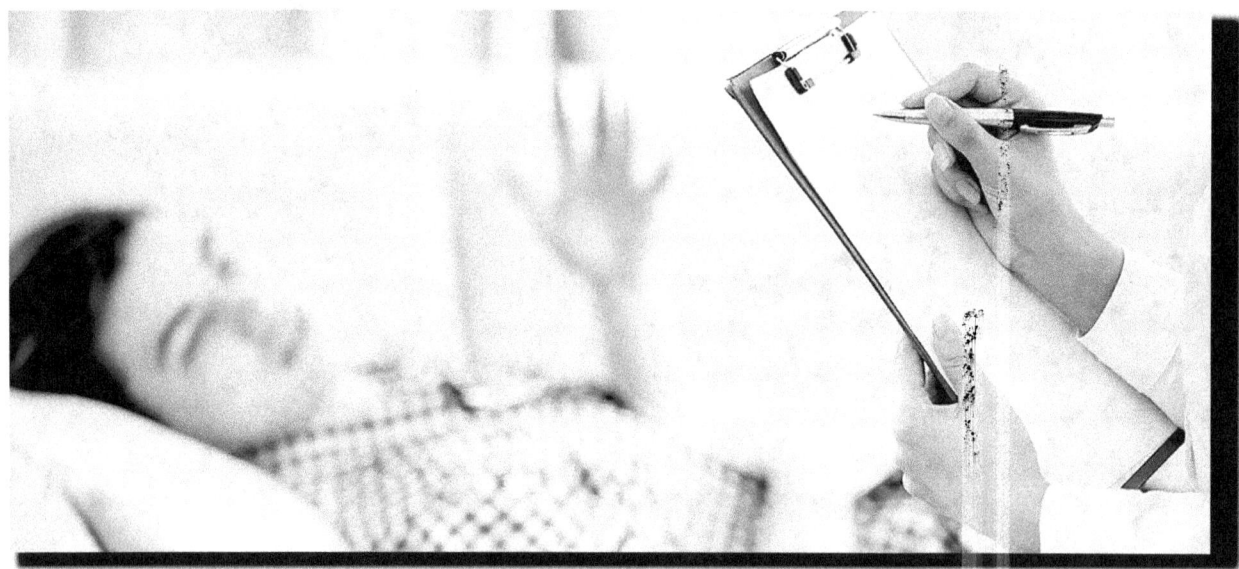

Child and Adolescent Inpatient

The Child and Adolescent Program provides intensive multidisciplinary inpatient treatment to seriously disturbed boys and girls, ranging from eight to eighteen years of age. Patients admitted to the Child and Adolescent Program typically have complex diagnoses, family problems, and systems of care issues.

A broad range of disorders may be treated but, in general, these are children and adolescents with disruptive behavior and mood disorders.

The average length of stay for patients in the Child and Adolescent Program is intended to be six months.

Psychology interns will participate with other treatment team members in the assessment of newly admitted patients and their parents, provide consultation to the treatment team regarding behavioral management, and function in the role of primary therapist for select patients.

In the role of primary therapists, psychology interns typically provide individual therapy, participate in family therapy and coordinate the efforts of other members of a multidisciplinary treatment team including direct care and nursing staff, child psychiatrists and child psychiatry residents, social workers, activity therapists, and special education teachers.

Psychology interns may also participate in and co-lead therapy groups and unit meetings.

Psychology interns will also be exposed to pharmacotherapy issues and assist the psychiatrists and the treatment team in the process of evaluating and potentially reducing the medical regimen of patients in the Child and Adolescent Program.

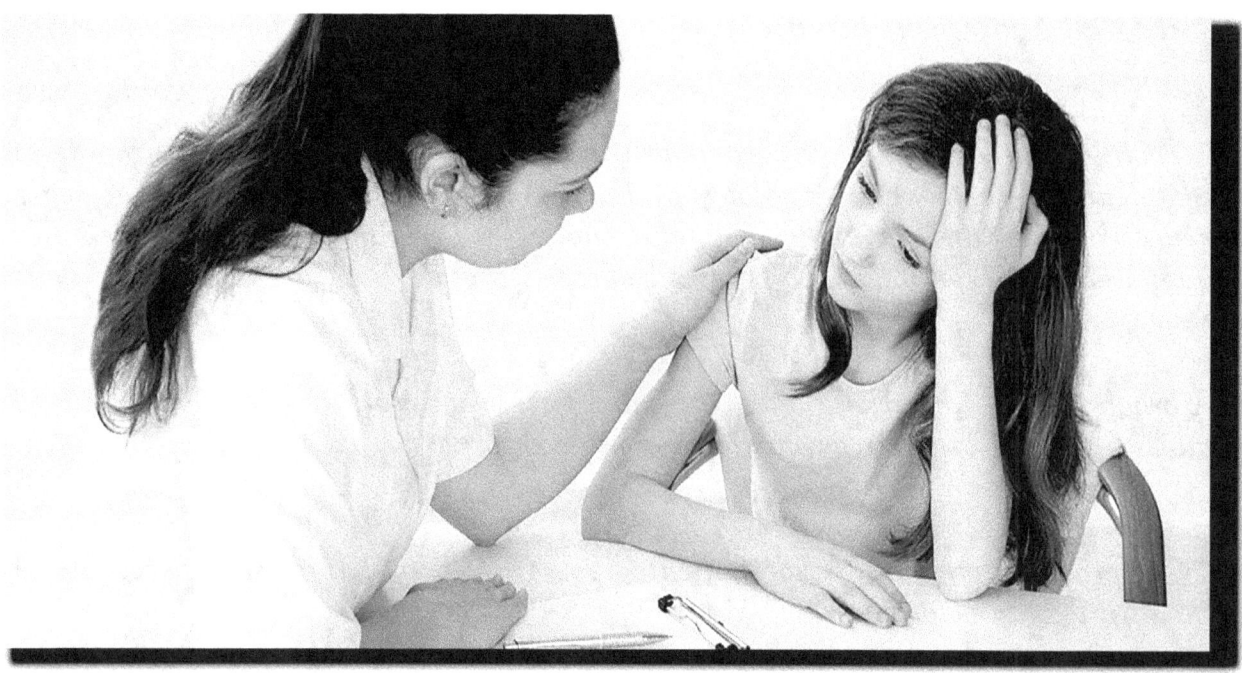

Child and Adolescent Outpatient

Psychiatry Clinic offers outpatient mental health services to families with children and adolescents under the age of 19. Families present to the clinic with a wide range of psychiatric and co-morbid medical conditions.

Specific experiences available on this rotation include participation in evidence-based mood and pain clinics, a full-day intensive testing clinic, and exposure to pediatric psychology.

Interns will gain experience working as part of a multidisciplinary team and will also have the opportunity to supervise psychology graduate students.

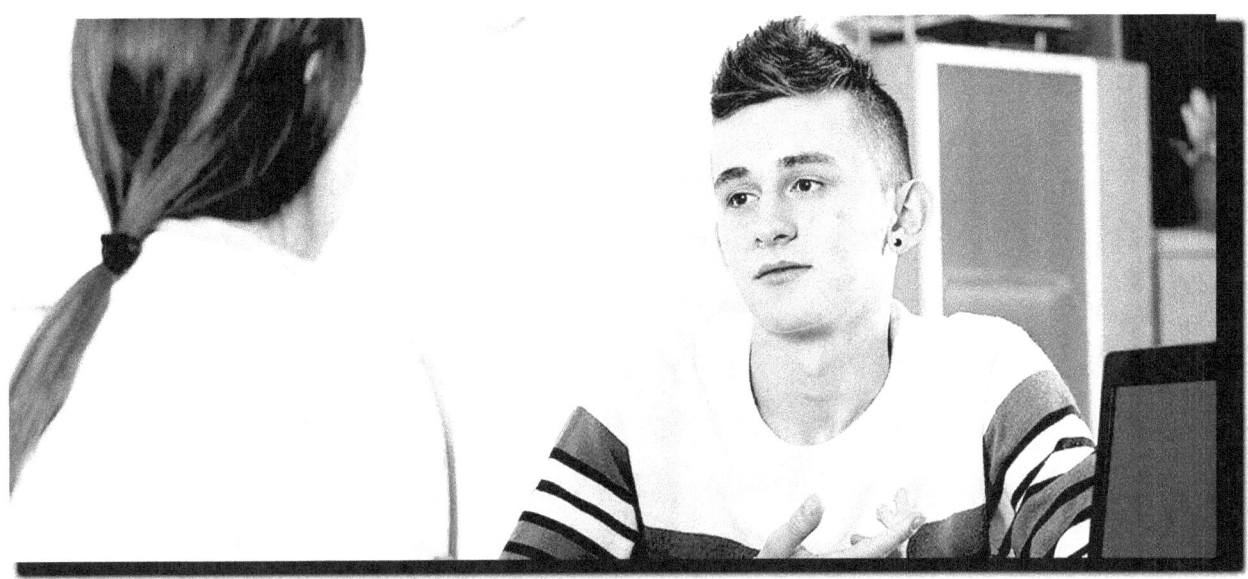

Autism Spectrum Disorders Outpatient

The Christian Sarkine Autism Treatment Center (CSATC) is a comprehensive, hospital-based and university-affiliated treatment center engaging in clinical care, research, education and outreach activities.

Psychology interns have the opportunity to participate in a variety of clinical opportunities that include both assessment and treatment of individuals with ASD. Assessment experience will include diagnostic interviews and standardized testing experiences.

The treatment focus of the CSATC is behavioral in nature with a specific emphasis on the science of Applied Behavior Analysis (ABA). Interns will carry therapy caseloads that will include multiple modalities (e.g., individual therapy, parent training), as well as a variety of presenting problems (e.g., aggression, self-injury, social skills deficits, adaptive skills training).

In addition to treatment experience, interns can pursue opportunities to expand their research skills on several ongoing studies based on time and interest.

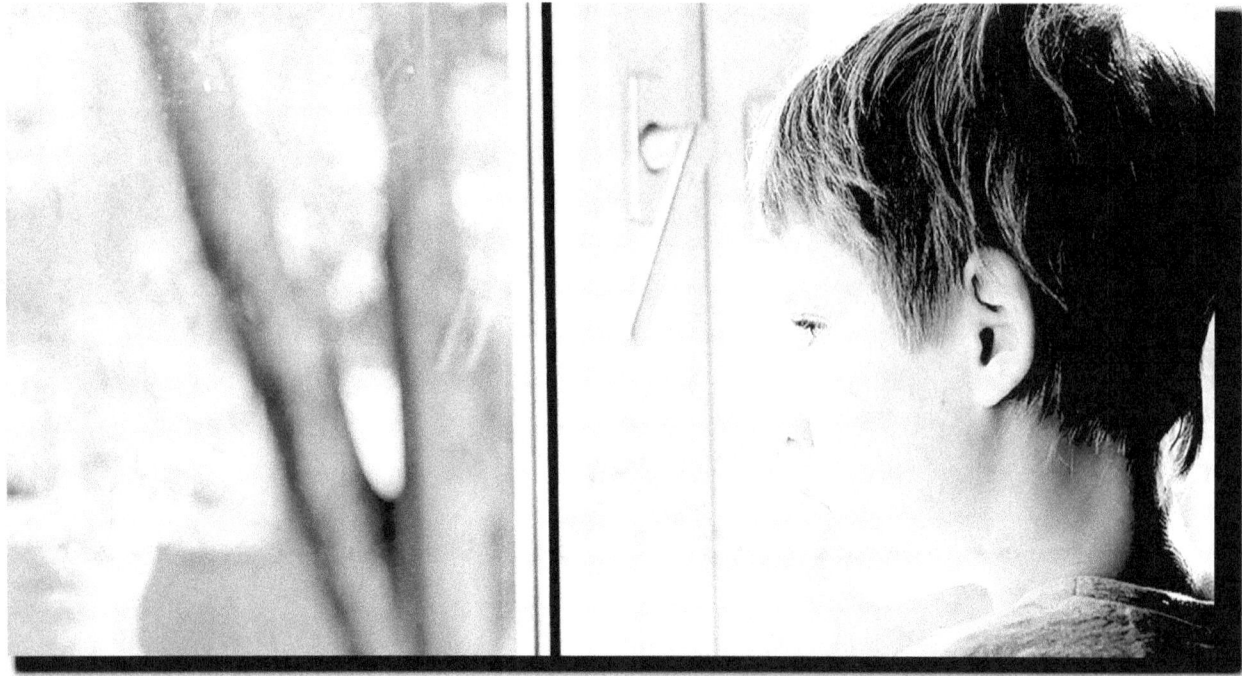

Specialty Rotations

The following is a list of specialty rotations that have been currently approved. Others are currently in development.

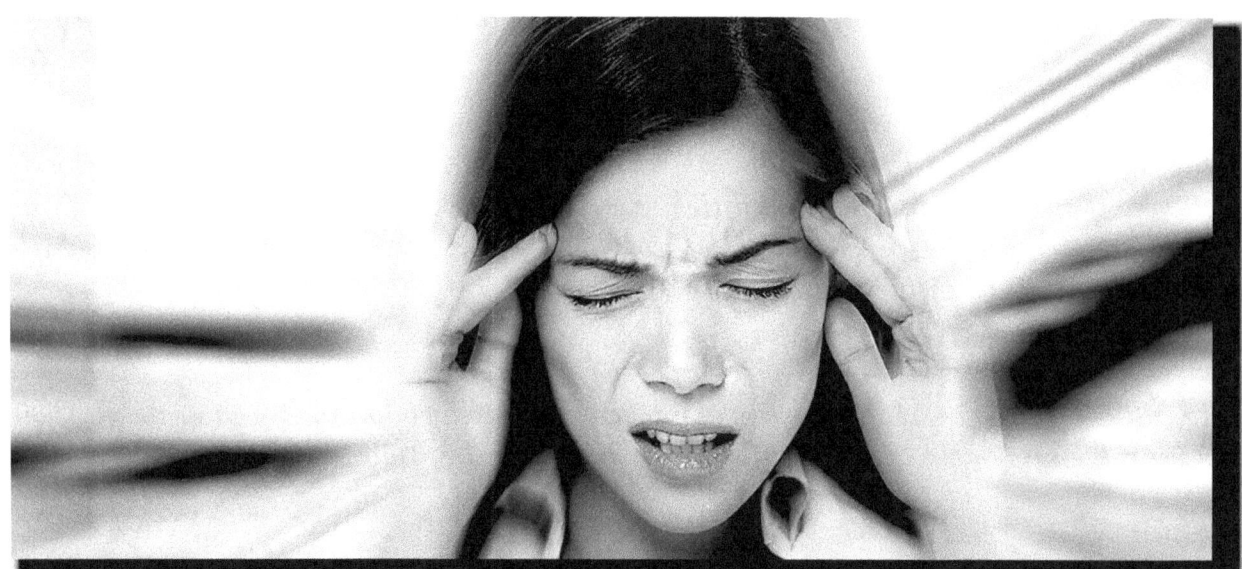

- *Pediatric Psychology Testing*
- *Child and Adolescent Mood Clinic*
- *Pediatric Overweight Education and Research (POWER)*
- *Autism Treatment Clinic*
- *Headache Clinic*
- *Pain Center Specialty Clinic*
- *Adult Neuropsychology*
- *Oncology Clinic*
- *Cardiac Clinic*

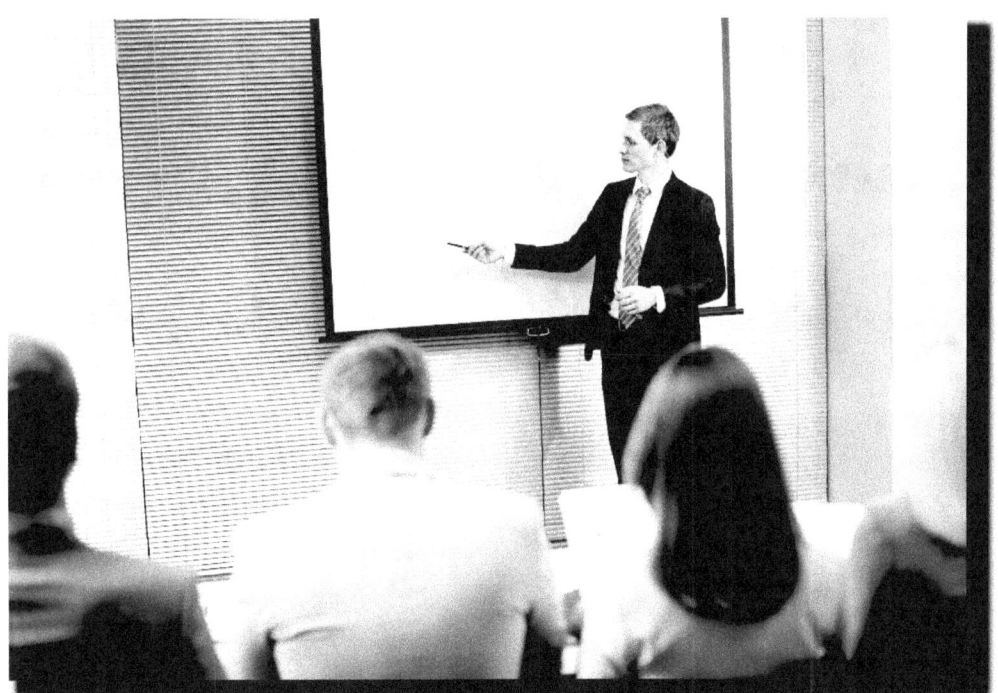

Para español vea nuestra

pagina web

http://semdcsa.com/es

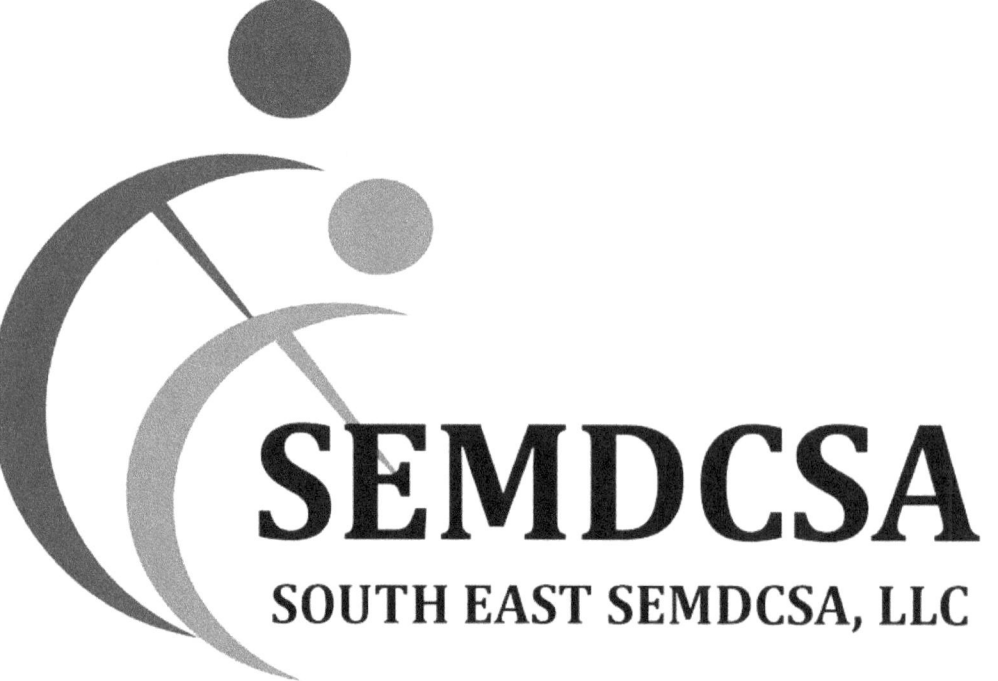

South East MD Clinical Skills Adviser   SEMDCSA   Dr. Hugo Romeu M.D.

34 | Page

REFERENCIAS

en Youtube

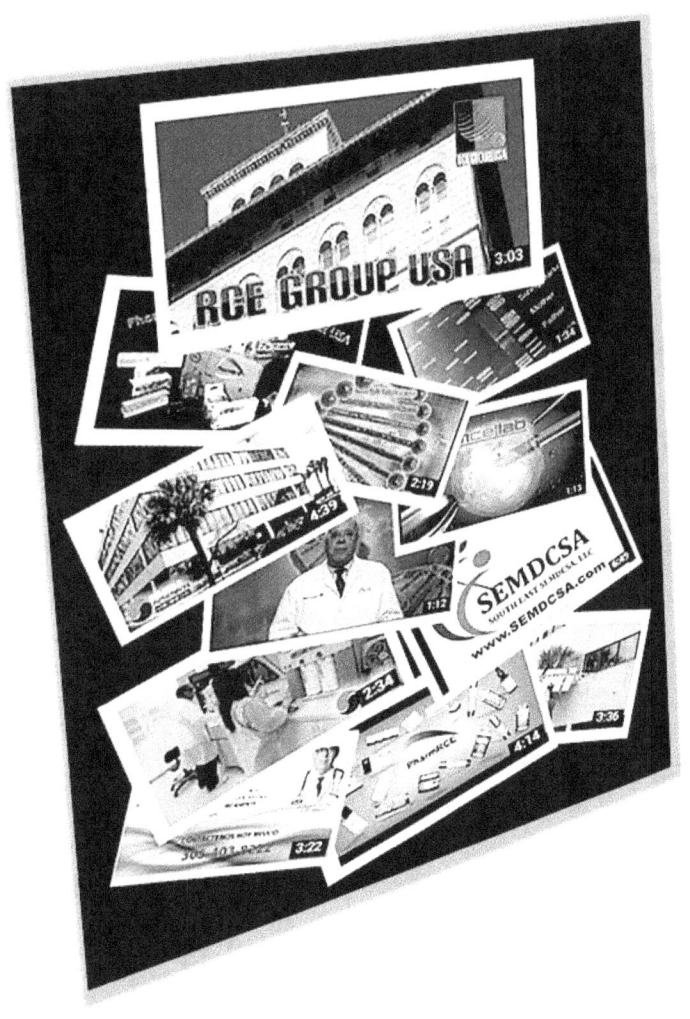

RCE Group USA

https://www.youtube.com/watch?v=BwkiIVehY1g

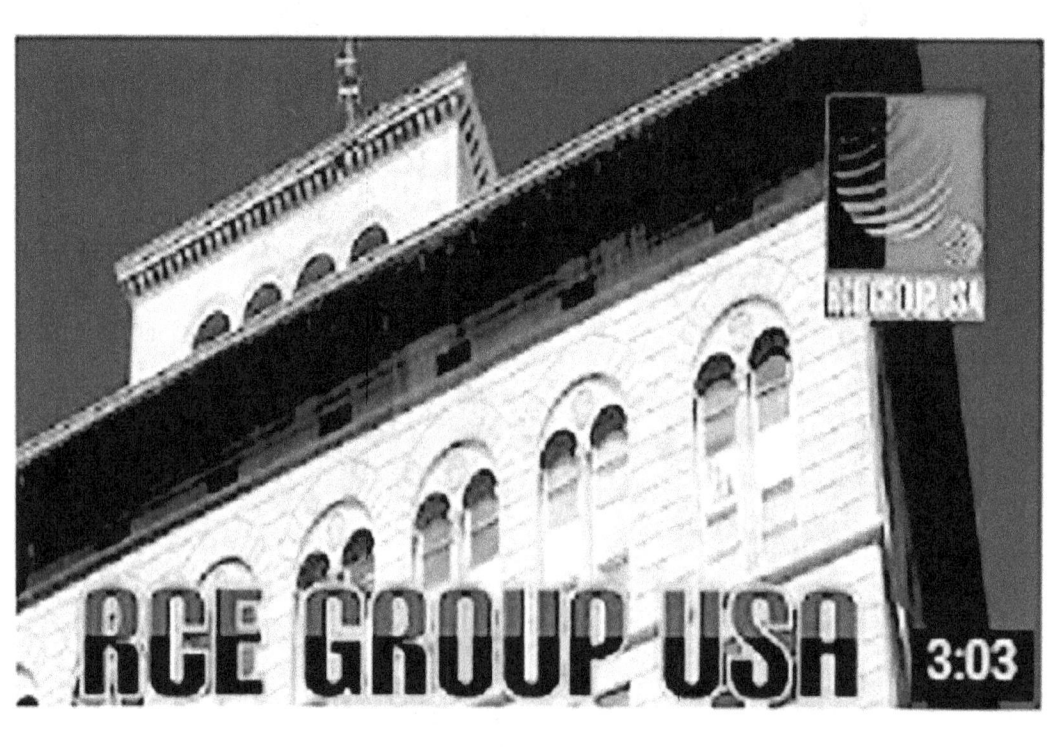

Reliable Research laboratory

https://www.youtube.com/watch?v=czvTqH5K-lg

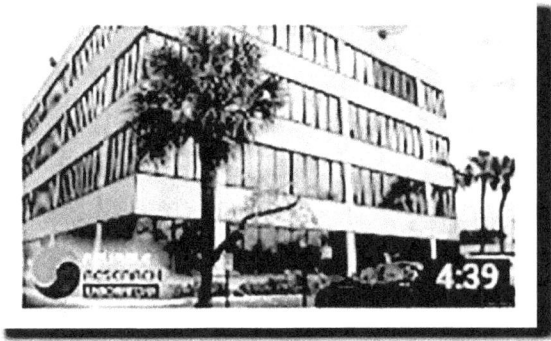

https://www.youtube.com/watch?v=2IYfrIaCkGU

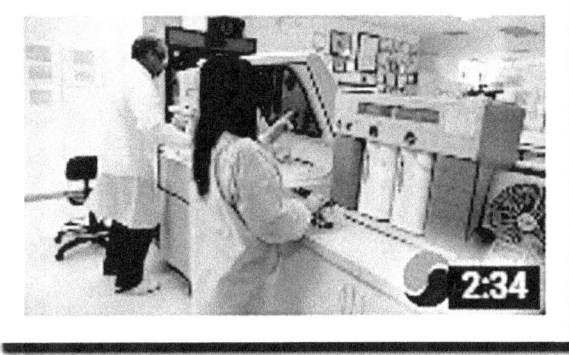

StemCell Miami

https://www.youtube.com/watch?v=UeygwgXr3vA

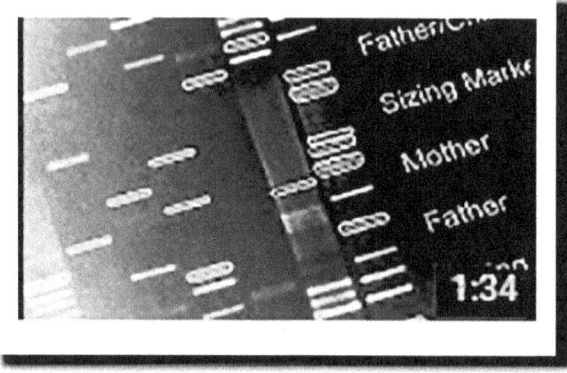

https://www.youtube.com/watch?v=QpBHg1EPvQs

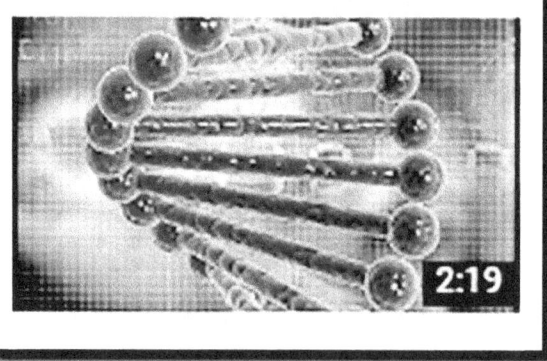

https://www.youtube.com/watch?v=xw4x_mV-RGk

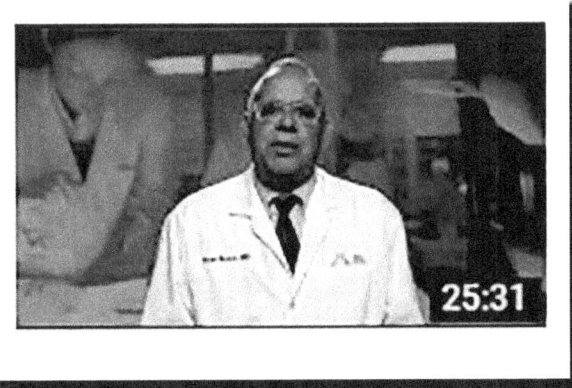

https://www.youtube.com/watch?v=Pa4LZdvoWc4

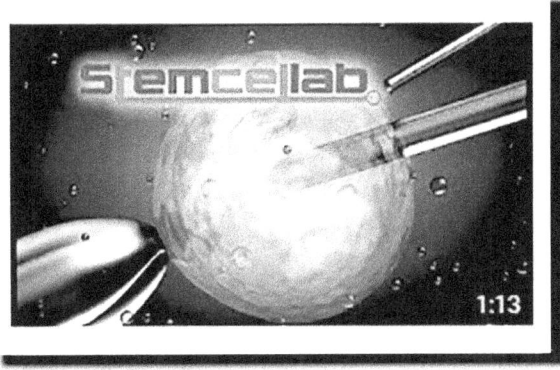

PHARM RCE

https://www.youtube.com/watch?v=dPpaXLpjU1o

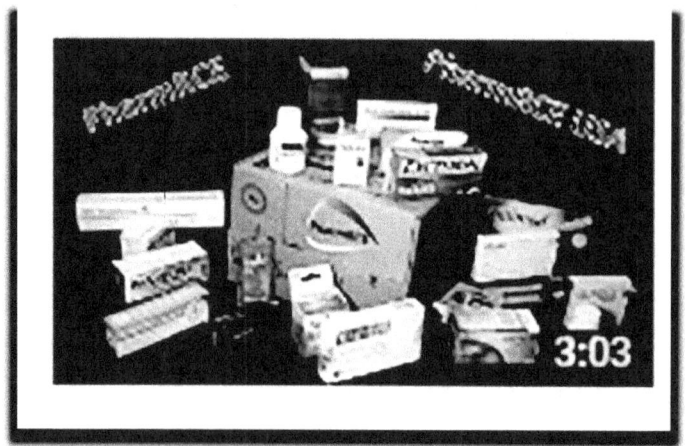

https://www.youtube.com/watch?v=pOaD5IpN70U

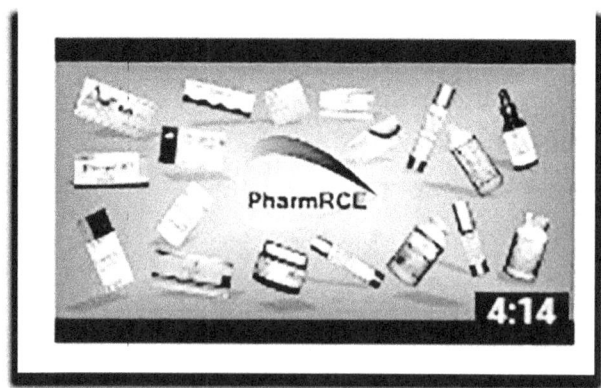

CRI PHASE 1

https://www.youtube.com/watch?v=HFNJiszSwTk

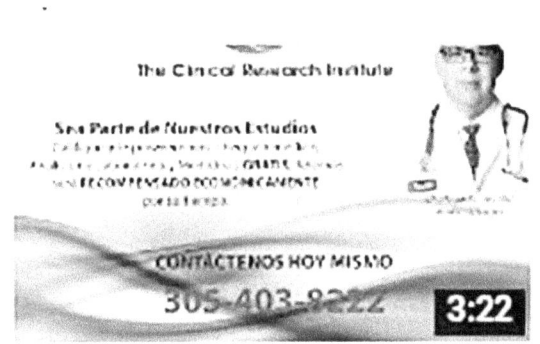

https://www.youtube.com/watch?v=1oRX6pYgZNU

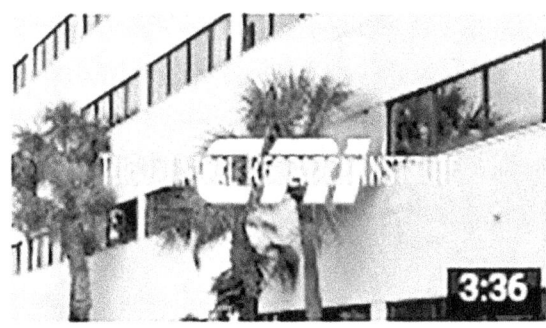

www.ingramcontent.com/pod-product-compliance
Lightning Source LLC
Chambersburg PA
CBHW080011210526
45170CB00015B/1972